SEASONS

My Journey Through the
Three Dimensions of Natural Healing

Beatrice Lydecker

Living Free Publications
15443 South Latourette Road, Oregon City, Oregon 97045

Table of Contents

Dedication

This book is dedicated to the many people who have stood by me during my illness and recovery, especially Deena Morando. She cared for me and my animals during the hard months when I had little or no money, and was too weak or disoriented to care for myself or them. I was very hard to live with then, and behaved irrationally as a result of my illness, so I am deeply grateful for her devotion. Without her, I don't know how we would have survived.

A very special thank you also goes to Mr. Richard Eamers of Los Angeles, California, who trusted me and believed in me enough to finance the start up of my company, Bea Lydecker's Naturals. Without his help, I could not have developed the formulas and products that saved my life and the lives of so many others. We all owe him a special debt of gratitude, and I dedicate this book to him with a deeply felt thank you for his care and trust.

I am also grateful to my pastor, Dr. Jack Hayford, and to his son-in-law, Dr. Scott Bauer, of The Church On The Way in Van Nuys, California. My spiritual guides and sources of encouragement and strength, they were the only Christian leaders willing to believe in me and accept what God was doing in my life. They often admitted that they didn't understand what God was doing, but they knew my heart and believed I was walking with the Lord. Without them, I am not sure I would have held on. Their teachings were, and continue to be, my greatest source of strength.

I am ever so grateful to Russel White, former owner of Cappseal, Inc., and to its new owners, all of whom for several years have patiently produced my product line. I will always be grateful to God that they believed in me, making it possible to provide my products, without interruption, when I didn't have the immediate funds to pay them. Never once have they cut quality, but continue to serve me faithfully. Without them, I don't know how I would have endured the hard times of the early growing years. They have been an endless source of information and support. Thank you gentlemen.

I want to thank my wonderful stepmother, Louise Lydecker, who, after the death of my birth mother, became my "mom" when I was a 13-year-old brat. She loved, supported and cared for me just as she did her own children. I am eternally grateful for the Christian ethics she and my dad instilled in me over the years, and for their unselfish labor of love by supporting me through Bible college. When, as an adult, I did things that were wrong, they continued to set godly examples by loving me while still upholding God's principles. They proved this by their comment, "We love you dear, but your actions cannot be tolerated in our home. When you choose to change, you are welcome back. But until then, you must leave." I knew I was loved in spite of what I did, yet I also knew that God's principles would stand firm in their home.

Included in my list of benefactors to whom I am deeply grateful are Bud and Georgia Basolo, two very dear and caring people who introduced me to the Herbal Extract. They realized that I was sick and convinced me to stay for a day to discuss how the extract could dissolve my tumors. I had previously spent many happy hours in their home swimming and playing with their wonderful gentle giants, Newfoundland dogs Charlie Girl and T-Bone. I also made their bulls very unhappy by performing acupuncture on them. The Basolos started me on the road to natural healing, which led from the Herbal Extract that saved my life to the development of the rest of my products that restored my health.

DEDICATION

So many more have supported my work throughout the years, freely sharing their ideas and encouragement. Some of these are the following:

Billie Kovacs, one of my closest friends, to whom I look as my Rock of Gibraltar.

Bill and Helen Thompson, my always faithful friends who saw me through many bad times. They were, and still are, consistently there to encourage me and help me pick up the pieces.

Dr. Thomas Abshier, who freely gave his time and knowledge to patiently explain diseases and processes that I didn't quite understand, and who took such good care of the patients I sent him.

My brothers Milnor and Richard Lydecker, and Milnor's wife, Sallie, and Richard's spouse, Joyce. My brothers believed in their little sister enough to financially aid me in starting my business.

John Byerly, who leased me my present property for so little, until I got established.

Lee and Bonnie Prince, who lovingly shared their property with me and my animals when I was homeless.

Lydia Hiby, who was my apprentice and cared for me and my animals during so much of the hard times. She was the first one I have trained extensively in animal communication, and she continues to make me proud of her accuracy and character.

Leslie Schmid, who always had a word of encouragement, and arranged many animal consultation groups to boost my income when I was trying to establish my local clientele.

Jackie and Marvin Happel, who opened their rental property to me with all my animals while I recuperated, and also helped me locate a permanent residence.

SEASONS

I have been blessed by many more supporters and encouragers along the way who are God's angels in disguise. May God richly bless each one of you.

Introduction

*S*easons may seem like an unusual title for this book, but one that I believe God gave me. *Seasons*, I think, best expresses the progression of growth and change in my life as I came to the point where I now stand. I borrowed the idea from the book of Genesis, in which God created the earth in stages. As I looked at these steps and at the lives of godly men and women in the Bible and in history, I recognized a pattern of growth and change as they learned to walk with the Lord.

The earth was not formed and finished in one day, nor do we advance from infancy to adulthood overnight. But as we *successfully* (and that is the key) complete each phase, we can then go on to our next "season."

We pass through stages of physical, emotional, mental and spiritual growth—the latter, in my estimation, being the most important. Anyone can grow physically, but too many of us get stuck in the wrong stages of emotional and mental growth. And far too few of us grow to the level of spiritual maturity that God desires for us.

Faith is a growth process, for as we get to know the Lord better and experience His hand in our lives, we grow to trust Him more and more. Faith is not easy, but is essential to every Christian's life.

This book is my journey of faith.

In *Seasons*, I will not reiterate my work with animals. This is fully documented in my two books, *What the Animals Tell Me* and *Stories the Animals Tell Me*, and in my videos, "You Too Can Talk to the Animals" and "Bea Lydecker Teaching Seminar."

Unfortunately, many in the Christian community have criticized my work with animals. Often, I was branded as occultish by those who do not know me or understand what I do. A tract

I've written, called "How to Cope With the Death of a Pet," was read and endorsed by Pastor Jack Hayford. That tract should assure its readers that I am in *no way* connected to the occult or New Age philosophies.

God has a purpose and calling for each of our lives, and we need to look to Him to know what that calling is. While I have been told to denounce and repent of my calling, *I will never denounce, deny or repent of God's calling on my life.* Rather, my heart's desire is to fulfill it. I was called to fit into God's plan for me, not to conform to what others think I should do.

Yet I feel so inadequate at times and often ask, "God, why me?" His answer is always the same: *Why not you?* You, too, will be surprised what God will do with your life if you will only trust Him and learn to listen to His voice. There are times we have no one else to look to for direction except Him. But as we grow in faith, we learn to respond in faith. Even so, God has given us living examples to follow in His Word.

When God told Abraham to leave his people (and go where?), Abraham went, even though God didn't tell him much until He got there. Later, after twenty-five years of waiting, God finally gave him the son He had promised. Then God told this loving father to offer his boy as a sacrifice—all the while promising to produce seed too numerous to count from that son! How many of us would have gone against logic and family opinion to do what Abraham did?

And how about Noah? Talk about faith! God told him to build a boat, load up the animals and his family, and sail on … what? He was on dry land way inland, and had no way to launch a boat that size. Yet he stood on God's word for one hundred years and built that boat, although it had never even rained before! How many of us would have lasted one year, much less one hundred years. But there was old Noah, faithful to God even though no rain was in sight and everyone was laughing at him (I'll bet they called it "Noah's folly").

The Word of God is full of examples of people who did not listen to man, but listened to God, against all odds and despite the jeers of others. The only difference between them and me is that they lived back then and didn't have the examples of great, godly men to inspire them. So their faith was even greater than mine.

We can be so quick to jump on the judgment wagon when people don't fit into the mainstream of society or we don't understand God's calling on their lives. Too often, we quickly brand them as eccentric, off-the-wall theologically, just plain wrong, or even satanic.

Aren't all believers children of God? Yes! And does He play favorites? No, I don't believe so. I believe He has chosen many to be great in Him, but they have not attained the place they should because they lack the faith to believe God in spite of circumstances.

I hear so many people say that God has called them to a great ministry that they look forward to someday experiencing. But what happens today? Do we faithfully put our hands to the plow and do the simple job God has given us to do TODAY? How many of us never reach that ultimate ministry because we've failed to complete our lesser tasks, fulfill our God-given seasons?

One of the most beautiful things I have come to understand about our Lord is that He calls us to a job for which He has already equipped us. He knew of my love for animals and gave me an earlier season caring for them, which has fulfilled and blessed me abundantly. And I will be eternally grateful that He has allowed me to continue enjoying a full life with my animals in this present season, which now focuses on working with people.

While I've long known that God was calling me to a healing ministry, earlier I thought He wanted me to be a Kathryn Kuhlman–type preacher. It took me twenty-one years to realize that He meant me to use my natural love of medicine to fulfill a healing ministry in a different way: healing with His provision found in nature.

That discovery and my work in natural healing is what this book is all about. I find this the most fulfilling, exciting task I could ever do. He has taken my natural love of medicine and turned it into LIFE for me and into healing for others. As Scripture tells us, "He formed [us] in the womb," and "We are fearfully and wonderfully made" (Psalm 139:13-14).

Thank you, God, for forming me as You have.
As imperfect and inadequate as I am,
with You I am in the majority.

Welcome to my journey of faith and discovery. I pray that you will find it as exciting and rewarding as I have.

He never said it would be *easy*. He only said it would be *worth it*.

What Happened?

The mist had hung heavily over the forest and left large dew drops on the leaves that glistened like diamonds as soft rays of sunlight shone through the trees. The fog outside seemed to match the one clouding my mind that even the hot coffee couldn't lift.

"Was I dreaming, or did I really see the big, round eyes of an elk staring at me through my living room window last night?" I wondered. "Or did I really see mink scrambling for cover when I opened the door to see what was stealing dog cookies from the Christmas wreath on my front porch?"

I wandered over to the kitchen window to watch the salmon struggling upstream to spawn in the crystal clear brook that quietly rippled past my trailer. To most people, this would seem like a paradise found. But for me, it was little comfort as I struggled to come to terms with why I was here on the coast of Oregon. Hidden away in the little town of Seaside, I lived in the middle of the woods seventy-five miles from Portland, the nearest large city.

For the first time in years, I felt a deep loneliness this holiday season. I missed my family on the East Coast, but most of all I missed the familiar surroundings of Los Angeles with all my wonderful friends and clients. I desperately longed for my church in Van Nuys, The Church On The Way, where I had always looked forward to and participated in the wonderful Christmas celebrations. My nearest acquaintances were my benefactors, Marvin and Jackie Happle, who provided this trailer in the woods until I could get my life back on track. But they lived so far away in Portland.

I never knew such despair. Here I was 48 years old and blown up to weigh more than 200 pounds. I used to run five miles a day, but gradually had become so weak that I could hardly walk across the room without collapsing. No matter how much I dieted, I just got heavier and heavier. My hair that didn't fall out had rapidly turned white. The pain that I suffered in nearly every joint and muscle left me exhausted, as though I'd been injected with a syringe that sucked out all my energy. Just going to the stable and spending one hour riding my horse, Feather—without cleaning or doing anything else—left me so exhausted I had to stop and nap on my way home to keep from falling asleep at the wheel. If not, once home I had to spend three hours in bed to even get enough energy to fix something to eat.

The candida rashes all over my body, especially on my feet, drove me to desperation. I had tried everything on the market to clear it, but to no avail. Just giving one consultation left me exhausted to the point of tears.

What was wrong? Doctors could only find a low-functioning thyroid, for which I took medication, and the Epstein-Barr virus. But they found nothing that should make me that sick. They told me it was between my ears, it was my imagination, it was menopause. Get over it and get on with your life. Yeah, easier said than done!

On top of everything else, I felt like I was losing my mind. I could set something down, turn around and forget where I had put it. Then I'd spend the next half-hour or more searching for what was right in front of me. If I had to run an errand, I'd often arrive at my destination and forget what I was doing there. I'd then drive up and down the street thinking, "I know I'm here for a reason, but I can't remember why." Often I'd pull over and pray until my mind cleared. But sometimes it didn't, so I would just go home.

WHAT HAPPENED?

In conversations, I kept repeating myself. But when some-one would tell me about it, I'd become uncontrollably angry with them, vowing that I had not said that before. When a checkout girl at the store asked me something or took too long, I became furious, yelling at the poor bewildered girl who had only tried to help. I knew what I was doing, but couldn't stop myself. I felt as though I was trapped inside a raving maniac. "I'm not like this!" I thought. "So why am I doing this?" Yet I was powerless to control it!

Tears spilled freely as I poured another cup of coffee and settled down to try to find some answers in the Bible. God was the only One to whom I could still cling for comfort. Only He knew what was wrong. As I cried out to Him, I suddenly heard a voice as clear as anything I'd ever heard say, *If you had not come away, in another year you would not be alive!*

Startled, I looked around to see if someone had come in, but the stillness hung heavy in the air. I asked. "Is that you God, or is this my imagination?" Again, the voice repeated the message. *If you had not come away, in another year you would not be alive!*

What did this mean? I knew I hadn't imagined the voice because it wasn't the way I would think. Besides, I'd heard that voice before. What had happened to bring me to the end of myself, and possibly to the end of my life? It would be another two years before I would fully understand and find my answers.

SECTION I

Seasons of My Life

Train up a child
in the way he should go,
and when he is old
he will not depart from it.

<small>PROVERBS 22:6</small>

Chapter 1

EARLY SPRING:
Planting Seeds

I was born July 12, 1938, in the town of Islip, in Long Island, New York, and was the last of eight children to John and Cornelia Lydecker. I already had five brothers, so everyone was overjoyed when a new girl appeared, or so I was told. My mom was already 45 years old and not looking forward to another child to raise, especially since she had diabetes and had her hands full with "the gang."

Satan has tried to kill me ever since I was born. At six months of age, I developed pneumonia and because antibiotics were not used much then, my parents bundled me up in heavy covers, opened the windows, and let the cold January air clear my lungs. It worked, and to this day, I love to sleep with the windows open with the cold air on my face.

My earliest memory is my dad trying to drive home by any new route he could find just to avoid the pony ring. There was no way he could pass one without my putting up such a squall he finally had to stop so I could have a ride. Horses and little girls seem to go hand in hand, and many of us know instinctively where the horses are.

When I was 5 years old, we moved to Bayshore, where we lived in an enormous house that was later turned into an inn. We had a little more money then, as Dad and my older siblings all worked at the defense plant during the war. Dad bought a boat, which enabled us to spend many hours of pleasure on Fire

Island. He always carried a big washtub for crabbing. My greatest thrill was when my family lowered that tub (with me in it) into the water and towed it behind the boat. I squealed with delight at that great adventure, the wind blowing through my wet, blond hair.

When we returned with a good catch of crabs, Mom filled the big metal tub with water, placed it over an open fire, and cooked those lively creatures. What a feast we enjoyed. It could be hazardous swimming in the bay, and more times than I care to mention, we ran into schools of those horrible, big round blobs of jellyfish. To this day I can still feel their sting.

I learned the greatest lesson of my life while living in Bayshore. It was a hard lesson, but I thank God for giving me the wonderful mother He did to teach me. One day when I was about 5 years old, I went to the store with my parents. It was just an old-fashioned dime store with an array of just about everything from kitchen goods to tools, but it was the toy department that interested me the most. I saw a doll I wanted, so I just picked it up and took it with me.

My mom didn't notice it until we got home. When she asked me where I got it, I told her. She promptly gave me a lesson on morality and stealing, and what it really meant to take something that didn't belong to you or that you hadn't paid for. She went to the big tree out back, broke off a switch, and proceeded to "apply psychology" to the back of my legs all the way back to the store, where I had to hand it to the manager and apologize for taking it.

It didn't make an impression on my legs because she didn't hit me that hard, but it sure did on my mind. She never hit me again—she didn't have to. Now some of you may call that abuse, but I call it a blessing. I still thank God for giving me a mother who believed in principles and honesty. I consider this a great heritage, although I didn't at the time.

When I started school in Bayshore, Long Island, I found studies came very easily. Their system promoted students to the next grade who could learn the full year's work in a half-year. But if you didn't learn, you weren't promoted at all. That is my earliest recollection of learning that work brought accomplishment and laziness got you nowhere—an ethic lost in today's educational system.

I loved learning and went from kindergarten through second grade in one and one-half years. I was just about to start the third when we moved to Salem in upper-state New York. They said I was too young to be in third grade, so they put me back in first grade, which was a great disappointment to me and a problem, for I'd already done the work. I developed lazy patterns for awhile, reading during class, not paying attention, and so on because I was too bored to listen. I guess I've never really forgiven that school for doing that to me, although I loved everything else about it, especially the music.

We had one of the world's greatest saxophonists, Sigmund Rasha, who made his home in Salem. He loved children and because I had a saxophone (only because my sister had it and we couldn't afford to buy any other instrument), he took a special interest in teaching me. It was a tenor sax, and if you know instruments at all, you'll know that was pretty big to a 7-year-old.

I remember sitting in a chair with my feet dangling, the sax in a stand beside me, as I learned the notes. He was a wonderful, patient teacher who gave me the best he had for five years. Those lessons and that music became the greatest joys of all my school years as I played in school bands, and in Sarasota, Florida, qualified for the Sailors Circus Band. When school got boring or times was lonely, I had that instrument to fill the hours and fill them I did.

We had moved to Salem to get away from the city and start a new life in the country. Dad bought a dairy farm, thinking my brothers would be there to help care for it. But my dad's lack of farming knowledge (he had been a city boy all of his life and knew nothing about cows) coupled with the fact that my brothers joined the military and left home, caused my dad to lose his shirt. Those were hard years for Mom and Dad, but there were some happy times, too.

My first skates were double-runners, tied to my boots. I don't know how much I "skated," but I do know I spent a lot of time falling on my keester with those things. I also tried my skill at skiing down the hill in the pasture. I never did get the hang of it, and rode those skies on my bottom more than on my feet. I've always admired people who could balance on skies for, even as an adult, I found it was an accomplishment to make it down a twenty-foot slope without sitting down.

In my adult life, I found it a lot more fun to go dog sledding while everyone else skied. I loved the animals. We had lots of them, too. I can still hear our guinea hens around the yard going "buckwheat, buckwheat" until we'd hear one say it in a high-pitched squeak. Then we knew that old Tom, our cat, had gotten another one. But one day, Tom disappeared. Dad never said what happened to that cat, but we didn't lose any more chickens or guinea hens.

We could sure create havoc sometimes, too, such as the day we were showing the kids our new baby goats, which got loose under the seats in the bus. What a time we had getting them out! The driver didn't appreciate it, but the children on the bus sure did.

We didn't have hay balers in those days—just a wagon drawn by a team of horses, a pitch fork, and me perched on top of the hay to pack it down as my family tossed it up. My brother John sure tried hard to help Dad with the farming when the other brothers left. But even he gave up when the team ran off with the hay wagon, throwing him under it. He was nearly killed when one of the horses stepped on him and ripped open his side. That was the end of my hay-stomping days, too, because they were afraid I'd get hurt. I sure missed it as I used to love to ride up there on that sweet-smelling, newly mown hay.

I loved those old farm horses. My brothers, especially Herrmann, loved riding them. They were tough, a lot of them being retired race horses. When my brothers hopped on them, they'd instantly take off. Once my brother Herrmann was thrown right over the head of one horse because it came to a crack in the road and, with no warning, stopped dead. Herrmann was in a coma for a long time, but that darn horse, which really belonged to our neighbors the Woodwards, would jump the fence and come over to our place to follow me around like a puppy. Yet he'd let no one else ride him.

We also had an old gray horse we called Smokey. He wouldn't go faster than a walk with me, and always went in one direction: up over the hill to our back pastures. I could pull until my arms fell off, but he'd go one speed and one direction only. When he got to the fence line at the back of our three hundred acres in the woods, I'd have to get off and walk him all the way home. He'd get me awfully mad, but I loved that old nag, and we were good friends until we left the farm and sold him to someone in Hudson Falls, where we would later live.

One day, my brother came to school to get me so I could go catch that ornery cuss. He'd gotten out and was having a ball all over everyone's yards, and no one could get near him except me. I sure felt like a traitor as he joyfully came running when he saw me. He was so happy. I turned him over to the new owner and, with tears streaming down my face, I left and never saw him again. I always wondered what happened to him and sure hope he had a good life. I look forward to seeing him again when I get to Heaven. Maybe this time, he'll give me a faster ride, since he doesn't have to baby-sit a little kid anymore.

My brother Richard (who is five years older than me) and I loved the spring because it was maple syrup time. Dad would hammer the spout into the maple tree to tap the new juice going to the leaves, which fed the new spring growth. We'd sneak out, steal the juice and drink it. It was so good. Dad would get so mad he'd like to choke us, but never did. We'd gather the buckets and take them down to the basement, where Mom would boil it down in huge vats until it was a rich, sweet syrup. Nothing tastes better than homemade maple syrup. I can still taste the sweetness as I savored the warm, sticky juice on Mom's hot, fluffy pancakes.

During the tenth and eleventh years of my life, there was a terrible outbreak of polio, and we were forbidden to swim in the ponds or lakes one summer. Many people became sick and ended up in iron lungs. Everyone was overjoyed when the Salk vaccine became available, and a great sigh of relief swept across America. When they came to our schools for mass inoculation, we lined up in the gymnasium to get our "polio shot." Little did any of us know that that shot would become as deadly to this nation as polio had been, just in a more subtle way, for it carried a potent monkey virus called Simian 40 (its effects are covered thoroughly in later chapters).

So our great blessing turned out to have a deadly sting, although we didn't have any problems at the time. All we kids knew was that we could go swimming again. In those days, we didn't get measles vaccinations either, so it was quite common for it to spread quickly through a school. When you came down with it, as I did, you had to spend about three weeks in a darkened room so you didn't damage your eyes. I was miserable. It was like confining a wild animal, for I seldom spent more than a few hours at a time inside. There was too much to see and do and discover in that big, outside world to loll around the house.

About that time, my brother Andrew came home with his wife, Helen. She was one of the most wonderful, loving and gentlest people I've ever known. She would spend hours talking to me, reading me stories and just trying to occupy me. They left shortly after my recovery. I was absolutely heartbroken. My mother was wonderful in so many ways, but we never really shared much. She was too busy taking care of so many of us as we didn't have the help of modern conveniences and appliances. We didn't get our first, hand-fed wringer washing machine until 1951. Laundry was done in the washtub on the kitchen stove. And all foods, such as breads, were made from scratch. So Mom had no time or energy left over to spend with an individual child. Besides, she was a very serious person.

But Helen knew how to nurture a child, how to laugh and have fun. Most of all, she'd read to me. I cried for days when she left. That loss affected me so deeply that I cannot help but cry now when I see a movie where someone loses a loved one or I see people leave someone they love. When I watched the movie "Shane," I cried for days over the scene in which Shane left and the little boy called and called for him to come back. The pain of losing Helen has never left me. My, what seeds we plant in our children without even knowing it.

Soon, she and my brother divorced and I never saw her again. She surely taught me how to love and nurture children, and I am eternally in her debt for that example. I would give anything to be able to sit down and visit with her again. My mother loved, but typical of the Dutch, she didn't know how to express that love in any way except caring for you physically. Hugging and cuddling is just not part of their culture. Later in life, Helen's example coupled with my love for the animals that demanded hugs and pets, helped me set aside my Dutch heritage and learn how to touch.

Thank you, God, for making up what we lack in our training so we can become whole human beings.

My fondest memories of my early life are our family outings. We were never allowed to work on Sunday, so after church we headed for Sunnyside Lake, where we spent the happiest days of my life. The Toomey family owned a pavilion with the first and only water slide I had ever seen. There was a small picnic area on the shore where Mom and Dad would set up the picnic table while we headed for the water.

That slide was only about thirty feet high, but it was awesome to us. We barely came out of the water long enough to eat, and back we went until we all looked like dried prunes, red and wrinkled. It didn't matter. We joyfully endured the agony of those sunburns. The delights and memories of family bonding and friends were worth every piece of skin we lost as it peeled.

Wonderful Fourth of July celebrations were also special times. That was back *before* patriotism, Americanism, love of the homeland, and pride in the American flag were considered dirty words and something to be ashamed of, as they have become today. The day started with the family heading for the parade route, with hours of cheering and waving the American flag. Then we'd head for Cottington's Custard Stand for a great big frozen custard. It's a form of soft ice cream with a taste that still makes me drool just thinking of it. My dream, when I am rich and can afford such a hobby, is to start a frozen custard stand and introduce the world to one of the greatest pallet-pleasers it will ever know—especially if you're an ice cream connoisseur, as I am. I'd sure like to know who invented ice cream as we know it in America, especially frozen custard. I think most Americans would like to join me in giving that person a ticker-tape parade!

Our day of celebration would end with everyone gathering at the school ball field for the greatest fireworks in the whole area (or at least we thought so). They usually weren't the grand explosions we see today. Mostly, they were patriotic designs, like American flags and such.

Years later, on July 4, 1996, I stood on the edge of the Potomac River in Washington, D.C., and watched the fireworks. There I saw buses driving by that honored the New World Order, instead of America. I looked across at the White House where, I believe, we have a president who no longer stands for America or morality, but who is a dishonest puppet of New World dictators who are stripping us of our freedoms and eroding all this country fought to build.

All I can do is cry. I wanted my girls to know at least a little of the taste of America that I knew, so I brought them here to see it while they still had the chance. But now I sit in grief, knowing that what we had will soon be gone. Such a far cry from the joys of family and love of country we all once knew. I will never be ashamed of what we were, and I'll do all I can, even unto death, to help preserve the Constitution that I love and the America that is my heritage.

One of the hard things about growing up so far out in the country was the lack of social skills learned with other girls. The only playmates I had from the time I was 5 until I was 12 was one girl at school named Betty (who was as much a tomboy as I), and Lyle Crosier, who lived a quarter of a mile from me. Because I grew up with boys, I just didn't understand girls and their silly, giggly ways. It affected my whole life relationships for I have always preferred the intellectual, no-nonsense conversation and company of men.

The guys taught me how to fight. You just didn't cry when you were down. You just got back on your feet and tried harder. So what if you had a scraped knee or broken bone, it was all part of life. You got up and went on, or you were called a sissy. To this day, it is still my motto, and what I am sure has made me strong enough to get through the difficult times in my life.

The other thing the boys taught me was how to meet a challenge. If someone says to me, "You can't do that," it is like waving a red flag in front of a bull. I have to prove I can. Built into my character, that tenacious spirit has enabled me to accomplish the things I have, in spite of the obstacles. Giving up was never an option in growing up, and I can never thank God enough for allowing me to be raised in that environment. The advantages have far outweighed the disadvantages, for the seeds planted back then have made it possible for me to keep getting back up on my feet through all the hard years of being knocked down. You'll understand that better, later on in this book. I still can't get into talking about the latest form of cleaner for tile and such. I would rather talk about politics, the latest medical research, new discoveries of any kind, and so on.

As I grew up, the only other girls I knew were the Sunshine Kids that came from New York City every summer. The state had a program whereby families in the country could host children from the city for two weeks every summer, and my parents always requested a girl. Since most of these girls enjoyed the country as something they had never experienced before, they stayed for at least a month. Those were great, fun times for all of us with a lot of tear shedding when they left.

Winters could sometimes be rough. There were days the school bus couldn't get down our road, so Dad had to hitch the horse to the sleigh and take us a mile down our dirt road to the Belcher store and the blacktop road to wait for the bus. We loved that because we would always beg a few pennies to get a candy called Shingles. Shaped like a shingle on a house roof, the candy was colored with three stripes and made of coconut. I've never seen them anyplace else, but if I ever do, my girls are going to get some. (I wonder if they will taste the same as when I was a kid?)

Whenever I go to the store now and see Entenmann's bakery goods, I always think of my brother Herrmann. He developed a special friendship with Willie, their son, when we lived in Bayshore, Long Island, as kids. He came to the farm for a visit and since our flush toilet was taking the pot to the outhouse and dumping it, he learned to use the outhouse like the rest of us. One day Willie sat on the outhouse seat, and no one saw the black widow spider that was there. The spider bit him, and before we could get him to a doctor, he began having convulsions. He nearly lost his life, and to this day my other brother Milnor, who also saw what happened, will absolutely freak when he sees a spider of any kind. I was afraid of them for a long time, too, and still exercise a great deal of caution when I see spiders until I know whether they are safe or not.

Being so far out in the country posed other problems for us kids at holiday times, such as Halloween. We were so far apart, it wasn't any fun going trick or treating. The only community nearby was Belcher, which consisted of about eight houses, most of which were populated by poor families with lots of children. Because they couldn't afford to give away candy, we celebrated with parties at our church. We never felt deprived because those parties were wonderful.

We did all the usual things, such as dunking for apples and scaring each other in the spook house by sticking our hands in cold, wet spaghetti "guts." Afterward came the great hayride, with an old team of farm horses that plodded along with steam billowing from their nostrils. With everyone wrapped up in warm blankets, songs rang through the night air until we finally got back to the church for hot chocolate and a bag of take-home candy.

Those were great memories of good, clean fun, but there were some mischief makers, in spite of the fact we lived in the country. Some of the older kids thought a church party was sissy, so they decided to make their own fun. I will never forget the time my brothers got together with their friends and decided to "make Halloween memorable for someone else, too." Since no one had indoor toilets, they decided to sneak down to Belcher and overturn outhouses. Now that wouldn't have been so bad, as the waste dropped into a hole below the outhouse, which didn't create a mess when the house itself was turned over. But the one they chose, unbeknownst to them, had a person sitting in it.

Just like any siblings, we had a great time watching our brothers "get it" from Dad, who normally wasn't a disciplinarian (in fact, they usually got away with murder). I don't recall what their punishment was, just what a delight it was seeing them get it. I don't think times have changed that much, just the pranks have. After we moved to the city, we went trick (which was usually soaping someone's windows) or treating. But that bag of candy we enjoyed never quite compared to the great church parties. Thank God no one ever thought of putting anything harmful in the candies. Back then, people seemed to treasure their children too much to do that.

Probably the biggest-deal event was to go to the movies. Like all little kids, I put up a terrible fuss if my brothers tried to go without me. When I was about 7 years old, the rage was the new Frankenstein and Zombie movies, which my brothers had to see with little sis tagging along. It made such an impression on my young subconscious mind that I could never again walk past the spot in the road where my dog was killed because I knew she would come back to get me. We don't realize how much we affect young children who are unable to distinguish truth from fiction, and expose them to so much that can change their lives forever.

No wonder Jesus wouldn't let the disciples chase the children away, but gathered them to Himself to teach and nurture them. A child is a delicate, precious gift. Handle it with care. Sometimes my family did just that, such as the time I became so angry with them that I packed a bag and ran away. My mom made me some sandwiches to take with me, telling me she loved me and didn't want me to go hungry. She wished me a happy journey and waved goodbye as I started down the road. I had no idea where I was going, but never made it past the spot on the road where my dog was killed. By dark, I was back on the porch, sitting dejectedly. When Mom asked me what happened, I said I thought I'd better wait until tomorrow and start out earlier, before it got so dark. She thought that was a good idea and invited me back in for the night. Of course, by the next day, it was all forgotten and she never brought it up again.

Gradually, each of my brothers either joined the military or married and left home, as did my sisters. Poor Dad. No matter how hard he tried, he just couldn't make the farm go by himself, so he finally sold it and we moved to Hudson Falls, New

31

York. The city was just what this action-starved country girl craved. I couldn't have been more excited to explore new horizons.

Chapter 2

CHANGES

When we lived in Hudson Falls, New York, my dad worked at the paper mill, as did many people in the tri-city area, for it was the big industry. I loved Hudson Falls. The best part of living in the city was that I had so many friends to play with. We could go to the store and, in winter, even had a pond to skate on that was maintained by the city.

The winters were exceptionally great, especially when the ice storms hit. We would spend the day skating all over town on the icy streets or challenging each other to a bike ride on the ice and snow. Every night I was at the ice-skating pond and, if I was gone too late, my brother Herrmann usually knew he would find me at the ice pond getting into a fight, defending some other kid (especially some little, helpless girl) from a foul-mouthed boy.

Even though I was a girl, I was usually winning when Herrmann would grab me by the back of the neck and drag me home. I think that secretly he thought it was funny but wouldn't let on, pretending that he was perturbed that he had to come out in the cold to get me. When the pond was melted, I headed for Brennans Roller Skating Rink with my best friends, Betty Merrill and Joan Wiley.

These were the happiest, most carefree and fun-filled three years of my life. The summer was wonderful, too. There was an old gravel pit about two blocks away that was loaded with pollywogs. We spent hours catching them in jars so we could watch them change into frogs. Now, if you've never chased pollywogs and watched them grow, you have really missed a special treat. I didn't even mind when I broke my finger playing baseball in the vacant lot, two houses over.

All my life, I had been an outdoor person, involved in anything to do with the animals, sports and work. When we weren't busy playing ball or sliding down the high mounds of sawdust at the sawmill behind the house, Mary Lou Munger and I headed for the stables to ride horseback.

The city provided unending pleasures to search out and explore. I was never home. As most kids do, I treasured my bike above all. It was my key to freedom, and when I thought I ran out of things to do, I'd ride it down to the river and fish. Sometimes I would ride my bike out in the country to South Hartford, to see my sister Martha, a journey of about ten miles. Mr. and Mrs. Smith and their wonderful Boston Terrier lived about halfway there, and always had a cool drink and time for a chat for this tired bike rider. They made me feel special, treating me like I was President of the United States and had honored them with my visit.

In the summer of 1949, I got my first job. Even though I was only 11 years old, I rode my bike three miles to Cottington's, where I cleaned motel rooms, hoed the garden, waited tables in the restaurant, and did general cleaning. At the end of each day, I was paid 75 cents and rewarded with a very large cone of frozen custard. I think I would have almost worked for free, just to get those wonderful cones each day.

I especially liked working there when the Sunshine Kids came. The only trouble was that they usually got a boy and ended up using him as free labor for the summer. None of us seemed to really care that this was wrong to do, we were just having a good time when we weren't working.

We always had a dog, even though my dad, at that time, hated dogs and cats. I guess my brother Milnor still hates animals because it reminded him of the farm, and he hated caring for them. It was easy to pick up Dad's attitudes, especially when we learned early in life that animals were not pets, but food.

While on the farm, it was nothing for them to slaughter a pig or cow for food, but what hurt the most was when they carried that attitude to my pets, our dog and cat. They just didn't believe they had feelings. Our dog, Spot, on the farm, had her litter of pups behind the stove, where it was warm, thanks to Mom's love of animals. We were usually able to find homes for them. But if we didn't, they were destroyed by shooting them. I suppose it was humane, as spaying dogs in those days was unheard of and we couldn't keep litter after litter ourselves, especially after we moved to the city.

One incident still haunts me. The pain today is as deep and real as it was back then. I was 12 years old, and Spot had had another litter. Dad wouldn't let her keep them because homes were scarce and since we lived in the city, he couldn't take them out and shoot them if we didn't place them. I had never seen what he did with them before, but this time, I did. He got a bucket of water and with Spot and me watching, put those pups in the water and drowned them. I'll never forget that sweet little mother, looking down into the water at her babies and looking up into my eyes, begging me to help her get them out. What grief in that dog's eyes, as she hung her head, followed my dad, watched him bury her dead babies and then lay for hours on their grave.

It wasn't long after this that Spot disappeared too, but they never told me what happened to her. Life was so cruel at times.

Whenever that picture flashes into my mind, I still cry for her and feel her pain afresh. Ignorance is such a terrible thing. We were taught animals didn't have feelings, so it didn't matter.

I think that has a lot to do with my insistence on spaying and neutering dogs that are mixed or who do not have responsible owners. I am not against professional breeders who take responsibility for what they produce, as I do, even to the point of taking back one of my breedings, a 12-year-old German Shepherd, because the owner didn't want to care for him any longer. I wish something could be done to stop this waste of life, the most precious of God's gifts any of us possess.

I know this incident still affects me, for if I see a movie about animals in pounds or anywhere being put to sleep, I still cannot stand the pain I feel and usually cry uncontrollably. Even to this day, I have to leave a movie such as "Dances With Wolves" because I can't handle the scene where they kill his wolf and horse. Why movie-makers feel they have to include such cruel incidents, I cannot understand. But I don't watch animal movies until I am sure these scenes are not in them. The seeds planted in my mind then still reap pain and care for animals, whereas the seeds planted in Milnor's mind still reap hatred and disgust for them.

My, how we affect others with our words, but mostly with our deeds. As the Bible states, "Train up a child in the way he should go, and when he is old, he will not depart from it." HOW TRUE! Unless God intervenes with a miracle or we see for ourselves what happens and want to change badly enough to make the effort to do so, we will suffer the consequences. I never realized how much influence our teachers have on our children until I became an adult and found out where my learning problem came from. In all the good things that happened in my childhood, one incident stands out that caused me grief and great struggles for years.

It occurred during my fifth grade. Until then, studying had been so easy that I spent most of my class time doing what I loved most: reading every library book about animals that I could get my hands on. One semester, I read more than thirty-five books, during classes, and still achieved good grades. There was another girl in my room (there were three classrooms of fifth graders) named Beatrice whose last name, coincidentally, also started with an "L." She was definitely the teacher's pet. When the grading period ended for the first semester, she had obtained the highest grade of any student in the three classes. Miss Shipey, our teacher, paraded her around to each room, bragged about her grades, and had everyone clap for her. I looked at her and thought, "I can do that too, easily, if I pay attention."

So I did. I put the library books up and listened. It didn't seem to make much difference. Instead it just made Miss Shipey mad enough to start doing hurtful things. I don't know if she just didn't like me because I was kind of a loner—a book-worm who lacked social skills and caught head lice every time I got near one. Or maybe she was retaliating for my lack of attention to her teaching in the past. During the spelling bees, whatever word I spelled, she always said it was wrong. Beatrice Larrow would stand up right after me, spell it the same way, and Miss Shipey praised her for spelling it correctly. I was stunned, to say the least.

When Valentine's Day came around, as kids still do, we gave out Valentine cards. Often we addressed our cards by first name only or by first name and first letter of the last name. Every card that read Beatrice or Beatrice L. was given to her, and I only received the ones marked with my full name. I remember looking at her huge pile (or at least it looked huge to me), and then looking at my little pile about one-quarter the size of hers and feeling very hurt.

Miss Shipey again had done it deliberately. This was not my imagination, as we all knew how she was. Even to this day at our class reunions, we talk about how mean she was to all the kids. We discuss how she would seat everyone according to what kind of grades they got on their report cards (the highest grades sat close to her and the lowest sat in the back). I wasn't the only one who felt her vindictive wrath, which only made me more determined than ever to get the top grade in all three fifth-grade classes.

When the semester ended, I was so proud that I had accomplished my goal. I knew now that my teacher would have to approve of me and praise me, too. So I excitedly took my report card to the front of the class to receive praise just as she had praised Beatrice Larrow.

When Miss Shipey looked up, I smiled and handed her my card. "Well, what do you want?" she asked sharply.

"Look," I replied, "I got the highest grade of all the students in the fifth grade!"

I will never forget the crushing blow I felt as she shoved the report card back to me and said, in a low, angry tone, "*Soooooooooooo!?!*" and went back to her papers, ignoring the crushed little girl who stood there fighting back tears.

From that day, my subconscious fed me the lie that to succeed was painful. For the rest of my schooling, including four years of college, I struggled to get C's. I barely made it through college, having to pore over books for days to learn what others grasped in hours.

No matter how hard I tried, I just couldn't remember it long enough to get good grades. It wasn't until I went to a marriage counselor, in my early 30s, that I discovered what had happened, and how my subconscious wouldn't let me succeed. It wasn't just in my education, but in my relationships, my marriage, or whatever I endeavored to do, I always found a way to fail.

A wonderful counselor at Narramore Christian Counseling Center in Rosemead, California, helped me work through the fear of success. I went back to college for a premed course and was delighted to learn I could again obtain A's and B's in the most difficult science courses. I'm grateful that I serve a loving God who didn't allow my life to be destroyed. Instead, He brought the healing I needed in time to turn my life around.

But wait! Let's get back to the story.

While living on Maple Street in Hudson Falls, God again intervened and prevented Satan's second attempt on my life. One cold, winter morning, I felt my brother shake me, and heard him call my name. It sounded so far away. My brain was so foggy, and I was so cold, I thought I was dreaming. I shrugged him off, but he persisted until finally, I woke up enough to allow him to pull me out of bed and shove me through the open window onto the porch roof. He then went on to rouse my sister and parents.

It was freezing outside, but the cool air began to clear my head. Soon the others joined me, and we gradually became aware that, had we gone undisturbed for another hour, the only thing anyone would have found in our house would have been bodies.

We quickly opened all the windows while Dad went to the basement to check the coal-burning furnace. He found that the flue was shut, which prevented the deadly coal gas from escaping outside. Instead, the gas went through the heater vents into the house.

Now, you may think that I'm a little paranoid, thinking that an accident was an attempt by the enemy of our soul, Satan, to kill me. But I have lived long enough to know his tactics. When the flue was checked by the furnace man, there was no known reason why it had closed. If my brother had been overcome as the rest of us, none of us would be here today.

Times were tough and money short, but we didn't know we were poor. My mother was very frugal, so we never went without the essentials. Finally, Dad was having such a tough time after he lost his job that we decided to move to a cheaper house in North Argyle, about ten miles out into the country.

Mom called it her "Little House by the Side of the Road." She had loved that poem, so she had it framed and hung in a prominent place by the door, to remind us of how fortunate we were to live there. It was fun living across from the country store, where all the locals got their garden tools, hardware, and just about everything else you could imagine—even a little food!

It was a small compensation for leaving the city life with all my friends. My greatest comfort was my horse. Dad bought me an old girl named Maggie. She and I had such great fun all summer. I learned every back road in the area, all the way from Argyle to my sister's house in South Hartford, seven miles away.

One day I wanted to fly my kite, but there wasn't any wind. I tried running across the field, but to no avail. I was suddenly struck with what I thought was a brilliant idea. If I got on Maggie and galloped across the field, I could create enough wind to get the kite airborne. Well, it was a good idea, but not workable. We started out great and the kite rose beautifully, until we neared the other end of the field. Then it took a sudden nose dive—you guessed it!—right in front of Maggie.

CHANGES

She quickly planted her feet and stopped, but I didn't. I was pretty sore for a few days but, thankfully, there were no broken bones. In the winter, I would saddle her, bundle myself up in heavy ski clothes, wrap the reins around the saddle horn, stuff my hands into my pockets, and off we'd go until we were both so cold and tired that we'd finally give up and go home.

For the first time, all my siblings were gone and Mom had a little more time for me. Her one great passion in life was her piano. She treasured that little spinet as though it were Fort Knox. She was quite an accomplished pianist, too, and could play for hours, song after song, from memory. She began teaching me the keyboard, instilling in me her great love of music.

I then got involved in an all-girl dance band, where I played the saxophone and sang. When we didn't have a pianist, she would pitch in and play for us. I believe those were the happiest times of her life. She smiled more than I had ever seen her smile before, and joined in with a gusto I didn't know she had. We only played for local granges and such, but those were times I still treasure. We spent many an hour playing together at home, too, just having fun with music.

It was hard for me to make friends, especially girl friends, as I had grown up in a world of brothers. My oldest sister, Martha, married when I was only a few years old, and my sister Florence moved in and out often. The one girl friend I did have, Pat Grant, lived about a half mile away. Even though we were friends and spent a lot of time at each other's houses, we were always in competition with each other in choir—but mostly for boyfriends.

My big crush was on a boy she really wanted and finally captured (funny, I can't even remember his name now). Well, I was heartbroken, as most 14-year-olds would be. When I was an adult, I went back to Hudson Falls to look her up and, sure enough, she had married that guy and had eight children.

I saw that man (whom I had thought I couldn't live without) sitting bare-chested while smoking and guzzling beer on the back porch of a rundown old house. He recognized me and yelled, "Hey, Pat! Beatty is here."

I was so shocked to see this "competitor" come strolling out, now at least 350 pounds, with half-naked children hanging on her skirt. When I left, I blessed her again and again for taking him away from me and prayed that God would make her life better as He had done for me. There's nothing wrong with having children or being overweight some, but this just wasn't the lifestyle for me.

I heard later that things did improve for her, except for the terrible loss of two of her teenagers who were struck by a car and killed while walking home from work. My heart goes out to her as I know she deeply loves her family.

All my life, I had attended church with my family. But back then, many schools also let out early one day each week, so children could attend a church of their choice for religious instruction. So my nephew Don and I attended Wednesday-afternoon Bible class.

People believed it was important to instill moral values in kids. I have to agree with them, for attending several different churches definitely enhanced my understanding of life, and taught me to respect different opinions and let go of what I didn't agree with. But we also learned moral values, something sorely missing from today's society.

I would often come home from school and find my mother on her knees, praying for each of her children. We knew she wasn't well from her diabetes, but had no idea she was as bad as we were soon to find out.

CHANGES

I had heard a lot of fire-and-brimstone sermons, where preachers try to scare you into Heaven. Now I'm sure that has worked with some, but not for me. The greatest change in my life took place with the arrival of an evangelist named Maurice Jacques. One night I attended a little church in Cossayuna, New York, and heard Rev. Jacques talk of a Jesus who left His glory in Heaven and set aside His power to suffer at the hands of His creation, man—even suffering a horrible death on the cross. And all this for me, so I could have my sins forgiven and live in a glorious place when I die. Well, I knew I wanted to know that kind of God, so I accepted Him as my Savior that night, and my life was changed forever.

When I got home, I could hardly wait to tell Mom the good news. She was sitting at the kitchen table, smiled the biggest smile I ever saw and said, "Now I can go in peace. I'm not afraid to leave you, now that you are in His hands. I know He'll take care of you."

That seemed like a strange statement. But to a 13-year-old experiencing the joy of having her sins forgiven, it kind of passed by as unnoticed. Little did I know that three days later, my world would change again.

The winters were cold in New York, often lingering long into spring. This was true that year, so we lived in the three downstairs rooms on one side of the house. Our living area was heated by an old woodstove in the dining room. My sleeping cot was situated between that old woodstove and my parents' bedroom.

That night, I heard a crash, and my dad yelled for me to hurry and come to help. I flew out of bed to discover that my mom had tried to sit up on the side of the bed and had fallen between the bed and the wall. Since she was a large woman, 5'9" and weighing about 250 pounds, he couldn't lift her alone.

When I reached her, she lifted her head, looked me in the eyes and quietly went home to be with the Lord she loved.

In those days, we didn't have paramedics or ambulances. It was the man from the funeral parlor who came to get her. They later told us that she must have really wanted to live as her blood vessels were so full of clots that they didn't understand how she could have lasted as long as she did.

Yet I know why. She wanted to be sure her "baby" was in the Kingdom and would be all right before she let go.

In those days, bodies were laid out in the home. So Mom was put in the front room, which was directly under my bedroom. It was a frightening time for me. I had never seen a dead body except in the horror movies. I just knew she was going to sit up at any time and start following me around.

Of course, nothing ever happened, except one small incident. I was looking at her one day when I saw the drape move, just below her hands. I called my father who reached in and pulled out Mom's little Chihuahua, Pee Wee, her devoted companion. The dog had somehow gotten into the casket and hidden by her side. It was hard to see the grief of that little dog as she was taken away from the only person she ever loved. I hope they are together again. If I know the God I know, I believe that they are, right along with ol' Spot.

A very strange phenomenon began to occur after Mom left us. As you entered the front door, the stairs leading to the two upstairs bedrooms were directly in front of you. My room was to the right of the stairs and opened to the attic. We didn't use the attic, so we put a heavy dresser and a large, old rolled-up rug in front of the door. There was nothing in that attic, but every morning, even though we never heard it happen, the rug and dresser were pushed back and the attic door was wide open. And this always happened after the footsteps.

CHANGES

Nothing ever touched me. But every night I was so frightened that I would crawl into bed, cover my head, and try to go to sleep quickly so I wouldn't hear or see anything. Mom had died at 2 a.m. and every night, at 2 a.m., we would hear footsteps start up the stairs, go up about five steps, and then fade out.

Everyone heard it, and even though we would stand quietly by the stairs, whether at the top or bottom, the instant we pulled the string that turned on the light, the sound stopped. Even my friends who spent the night heard it and would never come back.

We didn't know it when we bought the house, but every family that lived there before us had a member of their family die. I understand that whatever happened there before hasn't happened to anyone else, thank God.

Those days were very hard on Dad. He had been married for thirty-five years and barely knew how to cook. Mom had always done everything for us—cooked, cleaned and handled the finances—so we were lost. My sister Florence and her son Don came home for awhile, which really helped. Don helped Dad through his initial loneliness by keeping him busy, chatting about everything and nothing at all with Grandpa.

During the months that followed, there was one light in my dark world: my sister-in-law Frances. We had a strong bond because we both adored animals. When I was a kid I loved it at her place. She had pet chickens, rabbits, and a raccoon, and she raised Pomeranians and Chihuahuas. I remember riding my horse to Fort Edward, where she lived about seven miles away, and on the return trip she rode her bike alongside me to be sure I got home safely. She was always there when I needed a friend, and I loved her for that. I don't know what I would have done without her during those bleak days.

During the summer of 1996, I visited her and her new husband. She hadn't changed. She was in her glory as I watched her walk around her little farm, a pigeon begging to be picked up, her dog by her side, and her steer grazing contentedly. She had gotten them to raise for food but wouldn't let her husband, Ed, kill them because she made pets of them, too. He just laughed about it, but wouldn't let her near another calf auction where she'd gotten them. He is so patient with her, and even let her raise an injured deer that insisted on sleeping on the bed and went outside only to go to the bathroom. No wonder I loved her so.

By the end of the summer after Mom's death, we began to attend the South Glens Falls Baptist Church, where I became acquainted with two girls named Marie and Yvonne Langworthy, and, boy, did we hit it off big time. They loved my dad and I loved their divorced mom.

They lived in a small apartment, over the laundry where she worked and struggled to keep food and shelter for them. She had had a bad experience in her marriage and wanted nothing to do with another man—but we three girls had other plans.

The three of us would connive ways to get their mom and my dad together. After church, we would "impose" upon Dad to give this poor, tired, hard-working lady a ride so she wouldn't have to walk that mile home across the river. When Dad had to attend a Union meeting or a Lions Club, I would suggest he ask Louise so he didn't have to go alone, just as friends, you know.

I'd alert Marie, so she'd be sure to get the phone when Dad called. Louise would whisper, "Tell him I'm not available. I can't go!" But Marie would hold the phone so he was sure to hear it and then she'd yell, "Hey, Mom, it's John on the phone! Since you aren't doing anything tomorrow night, he wants to ask you something."

Louise would get so mad at us, but she had to take the phone or be rude, and she just wasn't a rude lady. Gradually, they got to know each other better, and spent more and more time together until finally Dad popped the question. By then, she was in love with him, too, so she accepted. There sure was some back-slapping, high-fives and rejoicing between the three of us over that.

But Dad felt, for some reason (maybe peculiar to his generation), that you were being disrespectful if you remarried before a year had passed after your spouse died. Because he didn't want me to change schools in the middle of the year, he and Louise bought a cute little house in Queensbury, and I moved in early with Louise and the girls.

That proved to be my dad's undoing, though. That winter, he was alone in North Argyle and struggling to keep up two houses (he finally sold one), then he was newly married and moving in with a new family. All that pressure and change caused him to have a nervous breakdown.

Poor Louise, here she was, a new bride, another teenager to care for, her husband in a hospital and with a house to pay for that her meager salary just didn't cover. But what a lady. She never abandoned any of us, but took it all on with everything she had in her.

When Dad got out of the hospital and finally came home, he had a long way to go toward recovery. His nerves were shot and his temper short, something I had never seen with him before. My brother Richard, a Marine, came home from his tour of duty in Korea and met my new 16-year-old sister, Marie. They promptly fell in love and married soon after because he had to leave for his next tour of duty.

The doctor recommended we get Dad to a warmer climate, so we sold the house, bought a two-bedroom travel trailer, and sold my horse to my neighbor, Barbara Hall. But the hardest thing I had to let go of was Mom's piano. It was treasured by the whole family, but we needed the money and it wouldn't fit in the trailer. Years later, we tried to buy it back, but they wouldn't part with it either. I don't blame them—although I would pay any price to get it back today.

Louise had a friend in Florida, so in the spring of 1953, we headed south.

Chapter 3

HEADING SOUTH

The trip south was rough. Louise, or Mom as I now called her, was afraid to drive while pulling a trailer. So Dad had to do it all, which was very stressful for him. Because he still wasn't well from his nervous breakdown, we had to stop time and time again while he took a walk to calm down (the way he had been taught to handle stress during his hospital stay).

It took a long time to get to Florida from upper-state New York. The super highways hadn't been built yet, so most of the roads were two lane, winding and slow. Pulling a trailer under those conditions only enabled us to average about thirty-five miles per hour.

The one thing that stands out the most on the trip was our nightly family devotions. We sat quietly while Dad or Mom read the Bible, and then everyone knelt to share in prayer time. They always acted as though our prayers were as important as their own, which made us feel like God was actually listening to us, too. No matter what our circumstances, those times, and my parents' strong faith and trust in God's loving care and provision, made us feel safe and secure.

It was hard leaving our families, but Louise never hesitated to do what she knew she had to do. Her new husband needed a warmer climate, so she simply moved us, no matter what the cost to herself. I've always admired her for that trait and still practice the same principle in my own life. She often said, "God never promised us an easy life. He just promised us that He'd always be there with us, and that it would be worth it."

Poor Louise. She always seemed to get the short end of the stick, as the expression goes. But I know that lady must be enjoying some wonderful rewards in Heaven right now. She deserves it. She built faith, honesty and character in us that is paying off in many ways that she never fully understood while here on earth—but I'm sure she does now that she's had a chat with Jesus.

She certainly lived 1 Corinthians 13: "Love bears all things, believes all things, hopes all things, endures all things. Love never fails ... For now we see in a mirror, dimly, but then face to face. Now I know in part, but then I shall know just as I also am known."

We don't always see the results of how we live, but like a rock dropped in a lake, we create ripples that go on and on. So goes the character she dropped into us. I am totally convinced that the people who make some of the greatest strides in life are those raised with principles and solid family lives such as I have experienced. Thank you, God, for giving me the mom and dad you did.

We were supposed to settle someplace near St. Petersburg, but plans fell through and we went south to Sarasota. Our first trailer park was on Siesta Key, next to the Stickney Point Bridge that went up and down with the passage of each boat. It was exciting to watch, and even more thrilling to come home from school every day and head for the beach or visit neighbors who loaded us up with oranges and grapefruit. Boy, did we enjoy that. Seeing those citrus trees heavy with fruit was wonderful to us Northerners. To this day, I don't think there is a sweeter fragrance anywhere than that of citrus trees in full bloom.

HEADING SOUTH

We ate so much citrus that we broke out in acid sores and acne all over, but we didn't mind. Those wonderful, sweet, juicy oranges were worth every blemish, especially since we were so poor. Dad's health and nerves never returned to normal, so he was only able to hold part-time or temporary jobs, such as a caretaker at the Jungle Gardens. That left us pretty short so, for a while, meal after meal, the only other food we ate was pancakes with a little sugar sprinkled on top, and tea, because we couldn't afford milk. Mom finally got a job working as a food-counter manager in Woolworth's, so she was able to bring home what we called feasts: food they hadn't been able to sell that day and couldn't be served the next day.

Later we moved to a trailer park in town and then moved on to Fruitville. Florida was hot, and when I say hot, I mean HOT. After growing up in the cool North, the change was welcome, until summer hit. We thought we'd die that first year and lived in wet bathing suits in front of fans.

Sarasota High was wonderful. We had Youth for Christ meetings and lots of band opportunities. At that time, Sarasota was the winter quarters for the Ringling Brothers Circus. So every year, the school put on what was called the Sailors Circus. I LOVED being in the circus band and still cherish my letter "S" with the clown's head inside. School was easy because they were a full year behind our New York school, so I'd already had the work.

Things went pretty well for us, but money was still very scarce. Finally, I went back to New York to live with my sister Florence so I could get better schooling in preparation for college the next year and to help make it financially easier for my parents.

I graduated in 1956 from South Glens Falls, New York. I went on to Columbia Bible College in Columbia, South

Carolina, to prepare for the mission field. Because I thought that God was leading me to be a missionary to orphaned children in South America, I concentrated on teaching courses and children's ministries. Those four years were good and bad, but my greatest joy was studying music and traveling with the college choir. If it hadn't been for the music, I know I wouldn't have lasted the four years.

I studied hard but suffered a lot from manic depression, found it hard to make friends, and struggled greatly with finances. If it hadn't been for financial assistance from my sister Florence, my brother Milnor, and for my parents' sacrificial giving, I would never had made it through. I had to work long hours in the kitchen to pay tuition, often doing my laundry, sheets included, by hand because I couldn't afford the washers. There I learned to walk by faith because God always came through with the necessities.

Eventually, it became evident that I couldn't afford to stay in the dorm because my long work hours were hurting my studies. So my parents moved to an apartment in state low-income housing, where many married students lived, to help me make it the last two years. This was a great sacrifice for them, but they wanted to make sure I graduated.

Mom worked at the Baptist Hospital as a nurses aide, which she loved. She adored caring for people, and took a personal interest in each one. I know she was a comfort to those hurting people since I saw many of them light up when she came into the room to care for them. She made them feel like she was their best friend, not like a nurse doing her duty to earn a paycheck. Although the money was vital to our existence, it was never about that to her. It was about people.

We were so grateful to Mr. Rossi who owned the Tropicana Juice Company in Bradenton, Florida. He was on the board of the Bible college, and every week he sent a semitrailer full of orange and grapefruit juice, which was distributed among all of us. I'm sure that got us safely through some bad cold seasons since there was no way we could have afforded to buy juice or vitamin C.

There were long lines, too, where we were able to get free butter, cheese and honey from the government. We were grateful for all of it. Dad was a carpenter, so he volunteered to help repair the roof of the church we attended, but nearly died when he fell off. After months in the hospital, he was finally able to walk with a cane, but was never able to go back to work again. Poor Mom. Again all the burden fell on her to provide for us—which she did, never balking.

One of the things that helped a lot was the hospital. They provided meals for their workers as well as a salary, so Mom got to eat well at work. One funny thing happened (which wasn't so funny at the time) that provided years of laughter and jokes for her and me until the day she went home to be with the Lord on Thanksgiving 1996.

It started the summer between my junior and senior year in college, when I traveled all over the South and Southwest with the Ambassador Choir from college. It was a wonderful experience I will never forget. But every church we visited for three straight weeks served us chicken for dinner in one form or another.

Well, we made it through that and when I got back to Columbia, Mom helped me get a job as a nurses aide at the Baptist Hospital where she worked. Someone had donated truckloads of chickens to the hospital so, for months, we had chicken EVERY DAY for our main meal. I never knew they could put chicken in that many different recipes. I have often wondered why someone didn't publish a cookbook called,

"Chicken, Every Way You Can and More." By the time that chicken was gone, neither of us could look a chicken in the face without gagging.

After graduation, I returned to Glens Falls to work and prepare for Nurses Training, while Mom, Dad and Yvonne returned to Florida. Because of all my years of working my way through high school and college without taking a vacation, I finally ended up in bed for a month with paralysis due to physical exhaustion. The winter was hard, so I headed back to Sarasota, where I got a job in a bank while I applied to mission boards.

Alas, I was no banker. I was constantly transposing figures, which messed up so many accounts they finally let me go. The mission boards turned me down because I was too "independent," too much a free thinker.

For a while, I tried working around town, but decent paying jobs just weren't to be had in those days. I lived with and took care of my voice teacher to pay for lessons. It was fun, and I did love the training and all the opportunities it opened for me to give concerts and substitute for the cantor at the Jewish Temple. It didn't pay a lot, but helped pay for lessons. She was an excellent voice teacher.

I tried out for the part of Maria in "The Sound of Music," which the Sarasota Players Theater was putting on. Sarasota is full of professionals who spend the winters or their retirement years basking on its beaches. So I was up against a lot of good competition. I won the part vocally, and even looked it because I am Dutch, but they were afraid I hadn't had enough experience to carry the lead, So they gave the part to a Broadway actress living in Sarasota. I had only had small singing and dancing parts in their previous production of "Carousel." Since there didn't seem to be much opportunity left there, I decided to go to California, where there were a lot of jobs and better pay.

Mom had a friend who lived in Orange, California, near Anaheim, so I decided to go there. I think I would have been on one of the first wagon trains heading West, had I lived back then. I don't know if I was brave or just stupid, but since I was always open to new adventures, I went. I didn't want to go alone, so I put an ad in the paper for another adventurer to join me. Roberta Aborn answered the ad, and off we went in a very old Chevrolet.

Chapter 4

FLOUNDERING

That trip was quite the adventure. We only made it about two hundred miles when our first problem's ugly head rose up and bit us: the generator had burned out. We stopped at an old garage on Route 19 where the mechanics stayed late into the night to get it repaired. We were so excited about heading to California that we didn't know we barely had enough money for gas and food, much less repairs. This had been our first adventure and, boy, were we naive.

When we left the garage, the guys stuck a flashlight under the car dash, and put a thermos full of coffee in the back. The thermos had their address on it, and they asked us to let them know if we made it—which we sure did. Years later, on one of my return trips home, I stopped by and again thanked them for their help. They still remembered us and were sure glad to see us.

After we got to New Orleans, we just had to see the French Quarters we'd heard so much about. It was interesting, but not what we expected. We stopped at Woolworth's for a bite to eat and some coffee. What a shock! The coffee was awful! It was the first and last time I'd ever taste chicory. I don't know how they could relish it so. Everybody in that area drank it. YUCK!

As though that weren't bad enough, we sat down in the middle of a racial sit-in demonstration. Since this was the first time I had encountered something like this, we were scared and couldn't exit quickly enough. We raced back to the car, only to find the car horn blaring so loudly you could hear it for blocks. We didn't know what to do until some guy came up, disconnected the battery cables to stop the horns, and then put them back on. He demanded $5 (a lot of money back then, probably equal to $50 now) from our meager purse.

When we complained that that was too much money for such a short job, he replied, "It ain't what you do, lady, it's what you know. Pay up."

That made a big hole, but we were two young, white girls alone in the middle of a black neighborhood, in a sit-in demonstration, with our car was blocked in, and all we wanted to do was get out of there. So we paid!

Our next problem was trying to get the car out. It was blocked good. And since I wasn't an experienced driver, we stood there, nearly in tears. A sweet black man walked up to us and told us he'd get us out. We handed him the keys, and he got in and tried to start the car, but didn't have much success moving it. We finally asked him if he'd ever driven a car like that, to which he replied, "Lady, I'm only trying to help you get out of here. I've never driven ANY car before much less one like this."

"What? You don't have a drivers license?" we asked.

"No, ma'am," he answered.

That did it. We would get out of there if I had to ram every car in my path to do it. The architecture in New Orleans may be interesting, but that was all as far as we were concerned. I got in that car and, to this day, I still don't know how we got out of that parking space. But by about four o'clock, we were heading northwest for Houston, Texas, where Roberta had some friends.

Although it was late, we decided to keep driving until we got there. Now, on today's major highways, that's not much of a drive. But back then, it was going to be an all-nighter. By nine o'clock, we were getting tired and hungry. So we stopped at a little café, in the middle of nowhere, surrounded by swamps in Cajun country. We'd sure heard some bad stories about Cajuns and how dangerous they were, so we were anxious to get out of there.

We ate, took NoDoz, and started out again at about 10 o'clock. We figured we'd get to Houston by early morning, find her friends, and get some sleep. But as we pulled out, the car's headlights got dimmer and dimmer. It was pitch black, so we crept back to the cafe. There were no open garages anywhere, so we had to wait until morning.

The cafe soon closed, we had no choice but to curl up in the car and try to doze a little. With all that NoDoz in us, you can imagine how much sleep we had that night. It was plenty cold, too. At the first light of dawn, we crept seventeen miles to the next town, where we learned that the bushings on the generator had burned out again. It cost $25 and took several hours to fix it. We were really running low on money now.

We limped into Houston bleary-eyed tired at about one o'clock that afternoon, but couldn't find Roberta's friends. We went to the police station to search some more, only to find out that they had moved away recently. You have never seen two more tired, frustrated, disappointed young women in your life. Remember, this was back in the days girls didn't make these kind of trips alone.

When we got back to the car, someone had let the air out of our tires. That was the last straw. We just sat there and bawled. Some benevolent, sweet man passing by saw our situation and returned with a pump. He looked like a guardian angel to us. Who knows? Maybe he was.

We made it about eleven miles west of Houston. We were hungry, exhausted to the bone, and filthy. But we were undaunted to make it to California. We noticed a sign advertising good lodging rates on the front of what appeared to be a private home. Meals, $1.50, double rooms, $11. Even if we went broke, we were ready to sleep on rocks if we had to. So we stopped.

"Meals" was an understatement. We each had the biggest steak we'd ever seen, and enjoyed all the trimmings. When they said Texas steaks were big, they weren't kidding. But we managed to get it all down. We went to our room, and each of us soaked in a deliciously warm tub of bubble bath. The beds had the softest feather mattresses I'd ever sunk into, and I think we fell asleep before we sank all the way down in those clouds of clean sheets and softness.

We slept twelve hours. A couple days later, we found some of Roberta's family in Lubbock, where we enjoyed a wonderful, home-cooked Thanksgiving dinner and a few days of rest and relaxation.

The rest of the trip was uneventful, except for the excitement of seeing the West for the first time. Since then, I have traveled America, literally dozens of times, and can tell you almost every out-of-the-way place to visit. Each time I take another trip, I always go a different route as far off the beaten path as possible.

America is a wonderful country with some incredible sights. Once, I hiked twelve miles to the bottom of the Grand Canyon and hiked back up the next day (I was so out of condition, I could hardly walk for days).

One week, I camped in my station wagon and explored every ghost town, dirt road or path in Death Valley looking for wild horses and Bighorn sheep. I enjoyed days of soaking in the hot mineral springs of Tonopah, Nevada. I explored the museums of Williams, Texas, the Oil Well Museum of Odessa, and the incredible museum in nearby Pecos.

FLOUNDERING

I've visited the hogans, chatted with the Indians in northern New Mexico, then drove for hours and hours through the wide open, desolate expanse of New Mexico, and watched the bats leave after I experienced the thrill of exploring the mighty caves of the Carlesbad Caverns. I've been enthralled by the wonders of the Cowboy Hall of Fame and those who founded our land after I shed tears at the Oklahoma bombing site.

There was the excitement of driving my motor home through New York City and then traveling on to Washington, D.C., where I experienced people of all nations as I watched the Fourth of July fireworks on the mall. There was the awesome power of Niagara Falls and the pageantry of Williamsburg, Virginia.

I recall my fun-filled days at Disneyworld and the Epcot Center in Florida. I've snapped pictures of buffalo while I watched the water spouts in Yellowstone National Park. Munched curds (that I begged from a cheese farmer) in rhythm with my feet as they crunched through the lava beds of Idaho as I searched for the river that goes underground and surfaces again where you least expect it.

I've appreciated the charm of Pioneer Village in Minden, Nebraska, as I walked through history in its buildings that house cars, farm equipment, medical and dental equipment, bicycles and much, much more, from the first ones made to the modern versions.

And I've cherished spending time at my favorite places in America: Valley Forge, Pennsylvania, and Tombstone and Bisbee, Arizona. You can just feel history with each step along the old wooden walkways or as you wander through the OK Corral.

Most of all, I've loved the people, the wonderful people of this nation with its varieties of accents and cultures, all blended

61

together to make up what I consider to be the greatest country in the world.

I've enjoyed the pampering of television studios where I was a guest on talk shows one day, and the next I visited the mountains of Kentucky where I met a charming, barefooted young girl with several children in tow. She looked over my motor home and dogs with the saddest, most longing look I've ever seen, and said, "I wisht Iah coud travel lake thaat. Iah got too many kiids. I jest keeps havin em, and don't know hauw to stop or whyy Iah kip havn em." The saddest part was that she really didn't know what *made* babies.

And I've loved the incredible ranchers with their solitary way of life on vast ranches as we rode on cattle drives. They loved the joke when this city gal didn't know that "mountain oysters" didn't come from mountain streams.

I've run with a housewife and felt her fear as we dove into a storm shelter to escape the tornado heading our way—a sight (and terrible roar!) I hope to never see or hear again.

I've visited the homes of some of the biggest stars in this country, only to find that they were ordinary people who shared a common bond with me: They loved their pets the same as I do.

There are those like the creep who overcharged us to stop the blowing horn. Then there are those like the generous men who cared enough to help two adventuresome, naive young girls by quietly putting a flashlight and thermos in their car.

There's the deep Southern accent of those folks who eat "Sardeeenahs" to those other folk who "paak caas" in Boston. But no matter how many countries I've visited around the world—and as great as their people are—I love America so much that I couldn't even bear to leave it to host my own daily television show in Canada.

FLOUNDERING

I would have returned to America probably pretty famous and definitely a lot wealthier, but I just couldn't do it. I love to visit other places, but I want to always be able to "Come Back Home."

California was a great experience for two young girls on their own. We immediately found good jobs and lots of great, eligible bachelors at the Marine base nearby. There was no end to the wonderful dates at Disneyland or standing out in our yard, watching the fireworks from there every night. In the evenings, our dates took us roller-skating or trekking around Knotts Berry Farm, which was free in those days. We went ballroom dancing all night at the Continental Club in North Hollywood, and then enjoyed the crowd as we all went out for breakfast before starting home to Orange. And we worked at the drive-in so we could watch all the latest movies for free.

Roberta and I took camping trips to inner Baja, Mexico, in search of adventure and of the lagoon where whales gave birth, and so much more.

Roberta found a husband, and I found a great job at the State Prison for Women in Chino. Many mornings, I had to be to work by 5:30 a.m., which put me on the road before daylight. When the fog got thick, I had to drive with the door open, watching the yellow line, so I'd stay on the road.

I floundered the following years since I had trained all my life to be a missionary to orphan children and, suddenly, I had no goal. I left prison work after six months because it was too depressing.

I tried teaching school, which I loved, but after a few years of that, I gave up. I guess I soured on that profession because they gave me all the classes no one else could handle because I had been a supervisor and group counselor at the prison. I handled them, but it robbed me of the joy of teaching.

I outsold almost everyone else in the Avon cosmetic organization, and went to manager training, but got bored waiting for an opening in my area. I helped my friends make ceramics to sell in their store, but that failed, so again I looked for another job.

Everything I did just didn't satisfy, or as soon as I succeeded and the challenge was gone, I got bored and went looking for something else. For twelve years, I traveled extensively and floundered around from job to job and relationship to relationship, mainly because of the unrest of my soul, not knowing where God wanted me.

The next few years were tumultuous, as my former boyfriend arrived in California and talked me into marriage. I went back to Florida, got married, and for the next nine years, lived in hell with an abusive spouse.

After my divorce, I started working with the animals, a great deal of which is related in my books, "What the Animals Tell Me" and "Stories the Animals Tell Me." I'll skip ahead to the time when those book left off, to my final arrival in North Hollywood, California.

No matter where I went, I usually ended up back in Southern California.

Chapter 5

HOMELESSNESS

M y health seemed to be pretty good. I'd been living in California in various spots around El Monte and Duarte. Traveling all over the United States and Canada in a camper van with my two cats, three German Shepherds, and one Pomeranian, I'd had speaking engagements for every group that would have me—from clubs of ten people to large assemblies in schools.

The first television show I did was in about 1969 with Regis Philbin, in which I talked with one of Johnny Carson's ex-wives and dog. From then on, articles about me and my work with animals started appearing in just about every major newspaper in America. Invitations also poured in for all kinds of media appearances from news stations to Letterman, Carson, Winfrey and so on. I started flying about 100,000 miles a year. It got so bad that my own animals would hardly talk to me when I came home because they were so angry I was gone so much.

Spiritually, it was very hard for me. I had trouble finding a church where I felt accepted until I found the North Hollywood Assembly of God Church. After driving back and forth between cities for so long, I was finally able to borrow enough money from my sister to buy my first home in North Hollywood. This home became a meeting place for our singles group swimming parties and dinners.

SEASONS

It was great being in the middle of everything that was happening. Every Christmas, I would spend days baking homemade breads, cheesecakes, and several turkeys with all the trimmings, for the open house I had for all my wonderful friends and clients. They stopped by to have dinner, visit and go on, leaving my home a lot richer than before they came. There were always at least seventy-five to one hundred people who came every year. (That's what I now miss the most in Oregon, for people just don't visit each other like they do in California. They don't seem to be very interested in being that sociable.)

I loved that house with its swimming pool. All of us enjoyed it, even the dogs. Someone brought a little pup they had found and asked me to find him a home. I thought he was a small, curly dog, but he kept growing and growing and growing until he became a seventy pound French Briard. He loved that pool more than any of us, and would lie by the hour on the top step, his long hair floating on the water surface while he snoozed.

I had a lovely foster daughter who, along with my nephew, lived with me for a while. By about 1975, I switched over to a Foursquare church in Van Nuys, The Church on the Way, which is led by Pastor Jack Hayford.

We would often don our roller skates to have a grand time skating the two miles to church and home again after services. Every evening, we had a great time running and playing with the dogs in the park. They looked forward to it as much as we did. They were hard years, but good ones.

As most people do, I had some puppies and ended up keeping one from each litter and pretty soon, with the German Shepherds I was also rescuing, I usually ended up having ten or twelve dogs in my house. Since animal control allowed only three, I was always hiding them.

HOMELESSNESS

One day, a Dr. Kutner came to the door in answer to my ad to place some of my dogs. He drove up in a new Cadillac with his wife (and young son?). He looked very weird. Dressed in a suit, he was wearing knives and two guns in holsters, which were strapped to his hips, cowboy style. When I called the police, they said it was legal, as long as the guns were in clear sight, not hidden. Anyone can wear them that way.

I think he may have been a plant from the animal control because the next day, ten minutes after I left with all but three dogs to go to the veterinarian, they showed up with a warrant to seize the extra dogs. But they only found the three, which was the legal limit. God was sure watching out for me. Since they aren't allowed to just come in, and we didn't have to reveal how many we had, the only way they could check was by looking over my back wall from the alley.

After that, I began to panic for fear of losing my animals. So the first chance I had to buy a kennel, I grabbed it. I didn't pray about it or ask God if this was His will for me; I just grabbed the first one I could find. They were, and still are, very scarce and overpriced in the Los Angeles basin.

It seems that most of my problems began when I bought the boarding kennel in El Monte, California. I called it World of Animals. It was in a terribly run-down condition, filthy with seventeen rats per three runs (we had one hundred and twenty runs, so you can imagine the problem). I brought in a lot of cats, but the rats were so big that the cats wouldn't challenge them. We got it somewhat under control as we cleaned it up.

I thought I could get it fixed up to board animals, and still be able to continue rescuing German Shepherds as a no-kill shelter. It would have worked if I'd had help, but the Shepherd people dumped dogs on me that they couldn't sell or didn't want because these dogs didn't turn out to be show dogs and other such reasons. But they didn't donate any money for their care.

They knew I wouldn't kill the dogs, but would keep them indefinitely until I found them homes. Instead of helping me care for them, they bailed dogs out of the pounds and other places where they knew they would be killed. I worked harder and harder to get enough money to buy them food, but alas, it took its toll on my health. In all the time I ran that shelter, I put to sleep only about ten dogs that we felt couldn't be retrained well enough to place.

So I started selling some of them to the military to raise money for spaying and neutering those that were going to homes. We couldn't get people to help buy food and pay vet bills, so I sold some to save others. I had been to the military base, and knew they were well cared for and happy to have a job to do. Doing animal rescue is like trying to empty the ocean with a bucket because people won't stop breeding and dumping pets they don't want or can't sell.

Until people realize animals have feelings, and quit treating them like disposable items or as a chance for their children to "see" babies being born (before dumping these pups at the pound), the pounds will remain full. Wonderful lesson they are teaching the children, isn't it? Sure wish they would let them see the pets being put to sleep, too, because there aren't enough homes for all those darling pups they watched being born.

Life is so dispensable to some people. If we don't like it anymore, just dump it—like throwaway kids, pets and families.

When I bought that kennel, I didn't know that it wasn't just run-down. It was also full of disease. Every dog I boarded went home sick, so I had to stop boarding. Every employee also suffered the same symptoms. After thirty dead dogs and $15,000 in vet bills, we found out that the grounds were infested with strongyle worms that we couldn't get rid of. All the dogs we were rescuing also were loaded with them.

When we started to clean up the place, another rescue dog would reinfest the grounds, and once the eggs are in the soil, you cannot clear it out. When I tried to notify the county veterinarian that the animals in the pounds were infested with strongyles, he threatened me if I dared tell anyone. The worms had mutated from horses, causing a disease called Strongyloidosis Stercoalis, which is still being misdiagnosed as Parvo, but is distinctly different.

Once I discovered what it was, we used Strongid-T liquid horse wormer, which got it stopped. Alas, it was too late. With all the losses and inability to open for business, I finally lost everything, including my $87,000 investment, and I had to file bankruptcy. The courts allowed the seller to repossess the kennel, so I ended up on the street.

I believe that the biggest contributor to my deteriorating health, and eight of my dogs getting cancer, was the weekly spraying of Malathion and other agents the state used to try to eradicate the medfly. It didn't work, but they kept on doing it anyway for three years. The kennels were mostly open, with pallets and doghouses, so they got the full blast of it.

These were extremely stressful years, too, and years of constant stress will destroy anyone's immune system. A lot of the animals coming in had kennel cough, mange and loads of fleas, so we used an awful lot of chemical sprays and dips, adding to our health problems. I later learned that everyone who had lived in my kennel and the one next door had developed cancer while living there, so I was just one in the long line. That place was polluted Big Time! I was burned out, too.

I had gained a lot of weight due to poor diet and stress. Because of the stress I lived under, I started drinking pretty heavily, too. An old swimming accident had caused a weakness in a disc in my back. With all my heavy work trying to clean and repair the place, and work to support it, the disc finally burst. I ended up needing back surgery, and also had two arm surgeries for carpal tunnel syndrome.

Bill and Helen Thompson, two very dear friends who had helped me retrain some of the dogs, came and moved my things to a storage unit. They also helped me move my eight dogs and myself into an old motor home. I headed back to Florida to recuperate with my family because, by this time, I had gotten pretty fat and was quite sick.

Since my animal work was established in California, I returned there nearly a year later to try to get another place and pick up the pieces of my life. But there just wasn't anyplace I could live with my animals. I couldn't bear to give them up, so I parked on the streets, in vacant lots and in the horse park in El Monte.

It was an extremely stressful time as the police were constantly harassing me, waking me up several times during the night to make me move. It was a pure nightmare until Bonnie and Lee Prince let me park out behind their warehouse on their five-acre grounds. It was fully fenced and they were grateful to have me because they were constantly being broken into.

I got a phone hooked up in their empty building and ran my business from there, trying to get enough money together to get another place. It was terribly hot. I was right on the railroad track with a factory next to me that spouted chemical exhaust. But at least I felt safe with three fenced-in acres for my dogs to run in at night.

But then some people in the old trailer park next door let the county know I was there. Again, the police came and chased me. The county said it was illegal to live in a motor home in a manufacturing zone. I couldn't win no matter what I did. One tragedy after another struck—animals were injured or killed because of the bad living conditions, and the police kept harassing me.

Finally, I was able to find a woman in the San Fernando area who was willing to share a place with me and all my animals until I could get on my feet. That went well for awhile, until the police discovered that I lived there. Because I had more than the allowed three dogs , I again had to move.

So I shared a house and expenses with Lydia Hiby in Redondo Beach, but again the police found out I was there, thanks to a pot-smoking neighbor who teased my dogs and, when they barked, called the police. The animal control again harassed me as they had in North Hollywood. They came around the back fence and made a lot of noise until the dogs went out to investigate, giving them the opportunity to count how many I had.

All the other neighbors went to court and asked that we be allowed to stay because we kept the place better than anyone who had lived there before. But the law said no. Apparently they preferred drug addicts to dogs. So again, I moved into my motor home to keep my dogs because I'd been warned that the animal control was coming to confiscate them. I escaped with only minutes to spare.

We then went to a kennel in Santa Ana that was for sale. With the help of a sweet lady in New York, I was able to raise $10,000 to put a down payment on it, and naively turned the money over to Ron Saffron. He was a longtime client I thought I knew, and was negotiating the purchase—or so I thought.

Three months later, I learned that he had pocketed the money and had never intended to buy the place. I was embezzled out of the money, and the police wouldn't help. They claimed that it was a civil matter, not a job for the bunco squad or fraud division, even though it was grand theft. I had no money to hire an attorney and couldn't find one to take it on contingency.

Once again, I was on the street, living in a very old, run-down motor home and had no place to go. I was totally distraught, my health was failing, and I was at my wits' end.

Through all this, I could have had it easy, but I just couldn't bear to part with my animals. I will be eternally grateful for Jack Hayford and his son-in-law Scott Bauer, for they were the only light and strength during that trying time. I went to The Church on the Way faithfully, no matter where I was living because it was the one place I found hope. Their faithful prayers held me up. They never criticized me but prayed for me and encouraged me all the way. I hung on their sermons as my lifeline because other than them, spiritually, I stood alone.

No other church or Christian organization would give me the time of day. Without even reading my tract, "How to Cope With the Death of a Pet" that Pastor Jack reviewed and endorsed, they all condemned me as occultish, shunning me because I was divorced and talked to animals and got answers.

Pastor Jack and Pastor Scott often told me they didn't understand what God was doing through me, but they knew my heart and stood behind me as a sister in Christ. They will never know how deeply I appreciated that, and the strength it gave me to keep on keeping on. I didn't fully understand it either—only that God had called me to what I was doing and I had to remain faithful to Him no matter what man said or did. It felt like God was either deaf, or couldn't or wouldn't help me. But I clung to my church like the spiritual life raft it was.

It seemed like it was going on for a long time and no let up was in sight. One sermon that meant a lot to me was Pastor

Jack's insights in the life of Joseph. For fourteen years, Joseph had served Pharaoh or spent time in prison. But there was a reason behind it. God was teaching him some important lessons and some character building was going on that was necessary in order to equip him for the tasks God had for him to fulfill.

I know that during that time for me, there were a lot of changes taking place in my heart and some valuable lessons I needed to learn. As hard as they were to suffer through, and I mean suffer, I am confident that it was for my own good to have to go through those trials. My God who loves me would never have made me endure what I did for no reason. I trust Him.

Another reason it took so long was my own fault. I knew God was leading me into a healing ministry, but I thought He was going to make me into a Kathryn Kuhlman, and there was no way I was going to be a preacher. When God finally broke me to the point that I was willing to do or be whatever He wanted, then things began to change.

Things also got bad because I think that God was trying to get me to move out of Los Angeles. But I couldn't bring myself to leave my beloved church and my beloved city where I felt so comfortable. I loved that area and couldn't imagine living any-place else. He had to push me to the limit, to make me let go, and be willing to move where He was sending me, which was to Oregon. Only then did the nightmare existence end.

By this time, I was getting very sick. I had gained sixty pounds, even though I was running sometimes five miles a day and dieting. My hair began to fall out and turn white, and my chronic fatigue got worse and worse. All the joy and vitality I had known through my life was gone, and all I wanted to do was lie down and die.

I had exhausted all the places I could find to live, and even the few friends who stuck by me couldn't help anymore because they were so overloaded with animals that they couldn't take any of mine. I was totally distraught. I had no place to live, my health was gone, and I was at my wits' end. I felt like Job in the Bible when he had been stripped of everything, even his children and his health. All that was spared was his life.

Then God used good clients of mine, Jackie and Marvin Happel in Portland, Oregon, to rescue me. They heard about my plight and invited me to come to Oregon. They had an extra mobile home in Seaside that was empty, so they invited me to I use it until I got on my feet. It was isolated, away from almost everyone, so with a breaking heart, my "heels dug in," and tears streaming down my face, I left my beloved Southern California for parts unknown.

Why didn't I go home to Florida? I couldn't stand the heat. And since I'd been in the Northwest and loved the climate, I went. This was a radical change, living seventy-five miles from town, in the woods. But it was exactly what I needed.

Chapter 6

GOD'S HAND AT WORK

I had plenty of time to think as I slept and rested away the longest, quietest and wettest winter I have ever spent. By spring, I knew I had to make a move because Seaside was just too remote for my work, so I started looking in the Portland area for a place where I could live safely with my animals. A friend of Jackie's introduced me to one of her tenants who had an available place just east of Portland in the small community of Barton.

The day we drove down the tree-lined, private lane and turned into the property, I knew I was home at last. I walked around the twenty acres, which were covered with a three-foot high blanket of blackberry bushes, weeds and grass, and had obviously been neglected for years. I felt a deep sense of peace as I prayed and claimed the land for our new home.

But how? I had no money and no way to get the $85,000 to buy it or the trailer that sat on the fifteen-foot high foundation. The basement was dirt, and open with nothing to stop the cold air from coming up through the unconnected, open floor vents into the mobile home above. We crawled up a plank that led to the front door and still—with so much to do to make it livable—I knew I was home.

When I contacted the bank that held the mortgage, I learned that the mobile home was in foreclosure. But they would allow me to assume the payments, which were low enough that even I could afford it. Mr. John Byerly was in the process of repossessing the land, but he was glad to have some-one on the property. So in April 1987, I moved in.

If it hadn't been for Mr. Byerly's kindness in making the land lease so low, there would have been no way 15443 South Latourette Road could have become my home. I only needed to come up with less than $400 a month to live, which was not a problem now that I was close to a city where I could find work.

Gradually the place took shape. The grass was cut back and Marv Happel put up secure fences and built stairs and a ramp (for my old dogs) so we could get in and out of the house. But my emotional healing took much longer. It had been so long since I had lived with my animals in a place I knew they were safe—where the police or animal control wouldn't come and try to take them. Every time I left for any length of time, I prayed almost constantly that God would protect them and the prop-erty. Then I'd rush home, fearing I'd find one of them injured or gone. It took a couple of years before I could leave with a sense of peace.

It wasn't that I didn't trust God—I did. But after being chased by animal control or the police for several years, it took me a long time to heal the deep scars of fear and pain. I pray to God that I never have to face that again.

God had intervened by providing a safe haven.

Two more precious friends are Victor and Carol Ives from Lake Oswego, who provided a place for me to park on their horse farm while the property opened up. They also helped with a vehicle and provided the opportunity to do a daily show at their radio station. The show was a whopping success and made it possible to reach new clients so I could earn an income.

GOD'S HAND AT WORK

By the time the station sold, I was strong enough to start traveling again. So God provided another wonderful client, Deena Morando, to live here and care for the animals while I was gone. I couldn't get the basement enclosed for the first couple of years, which left the downstairs water pipes exposed to one of the coldest winters in Oregon's history. When they burst, poor Deena had to haul water for all the animals until my good friends Dave and Sharon Roe could get there to replace the pipes and enclose the basement to prevent it from happening again.

I don't know what we would have done without them because I didn't have the money to hire it done. Again, God intervened to protect and provide for us. They were, and still are, my angels in disguise.

Because I was so well established in Southern California, I spent one week a month at the Holistic Animal Clinic in North Hollywood consulting with people and their pets. They were hard trips, but the motor home made them economically feasible. I took a few dogs each trip for company and protection, and my dear friends Bill and Helen Thompson provided a place to park. But my greatest joy of the whole trip were the two weekends I had a month at my beloved The Church On The Way. At least part of the time, I felt as though I were going home to familiar surroundings and friends. And I knew that my animals were in a safe place and with someone who cared deeply about them.

Thank you, Deena, for loving my animals.

In the fall of 1989, I was to experience the Hand of God on my life in a way I never could have imagined. I had just completed my week at the Holistic Animal Clinic, but before heading home, decided to make one last trip to San Diego to do a horse group. I noticed that I was feeling more tired than usual, but just chalked it up to the twenty-plus horses I'd talked to on top of a busy week. The pain that had started in my stomach that morning was intensifying and my stools were black, tarry and more than usual, but I still didn't think anything was wrong. Since it was getting late, I decided to stay the night at the stable and head home Sunday morning. God had other plans.

The day started with the usual warm Southern California sun and temperatures above normal for just a few days before Thanksgiving. There was still time to make it to church, so I put the key into the ignition, put my motor home in gear and sat there, revving the engine but going nowhere. I was frustrated because I was anxious to get home for the holiday, but no one on the place knew what to do, so there I sat.

I thought this was an attack of Satan so I sat there binding him, commanding him to get away from my vehicle. Now this had worked at other times and, miraculously, things straightened out. But not this time. I just sat there.

In the afternoon, one of the horse riders came by to chat. He was a mechanic who happily took a look under the hood. He discovered that a special belt that extended to the second exhaust fan had broken and needed to be replaced. He couldn't do it, but knew someone who could. A couple of phone calls later, he informed me it would be Monday before they could get the part. "Sorry," he said, leaving a dejected, lonely woman sitting with her dogs on the steps of a motor home. All I could do was sleep and rest for the trip home. But since I am not one to take setbacks calmly, I fumed and fussed. Little good it did me; it just made matters worse.

Bright and early Monday morning, the mechanic came by and repaired the break, but things kept delaying me. It was almost like something was holding me back so that it was nearly evening before I pulled out of there and headed north. Since it was so late when I hit the San Fernando Valley, I decided to stay with Bill and Helen and head north into the San Juaquin Valley the next day, one of the loneliest and (at that time) longest, most-deserted stretches of Interstate-5 between San Diego and Canada. There were sometimes nearly a hundred miles between gas stations, and towns were nearly nonexistent.

On Tuesday I woke early, but felt so weak I could hardly get going. When I stepped out of the shower, I noticed how bloated I looked, my skin was nearly gray and, in spite of the cool air, I was sweating. The pain in my stomach had become so intense that I couldn't eat. I just sipped on a hot cup of coffee, downed a couple of aspirins, and resolved even more than ever to get going and get back to Oregon.

It was nearly noon when I had finally loaded up the dogs and me, but I just couldn't leave. I heard that same inner voice tell me, *Get to the Holistic Clinic—Now!* Since I'd learned to listen to that voice, I didn't head north to the valley, but went back to the clinic. When I walked in, I felt like everything I had consumed in the last month was about to come out both ends.

Dr. John Ottaviano had been wandering around the clinic mumbling, "I need to be out of here, but I just can't leave. I don't know why. I'm late for my lunch hour and, even though I have nothing to do here, I can't leave!" None of us knew why, but God did. The doctor took one look at me and said, "Bea, what's the matter? You look like you're in shock! Sit down and let me check you!"

I had barely hit the chair when I started throwing up copious amounts of blood. The attendants carried me to the table where I felt a slight bump and the next thing I knew, I was

79

standing beside my body watching Dr. Ottaviano work on me. He yelled, "Call 911, I can't get a pulse!" Then he inserted acupuncture needles in the heart stimulation points.

The next thing I knew, I was back in my body and waking up as the paramedics gently shook me. The clinic attendants took my friends' phone number and called to ask them to come and get my animals and the motor home.

The last thing I remember was the stretcher being loaded into the ambulance and then waking up in the hospital emergency room. Jack Hayford Jr. met me there and, while he prayed for me, I again passed out.

I spent the next five days in intensive care. But by Thanksgiving, I was in a regular room and sipping jello, which I pretended was a delicious Turkey dinner. That only lasted a few hours, for by evening I again started throwing up blood, and my blood pressure dropped so low that it was nearly undetectable. With three IVs going full out, the hospital staff wheeled me back to intensive care and called in the doctor to cauterize the hole in my stomach.

The room was quiet except for the nurse checking me every few minutes while we waited. I looked down and, much to my surprise, I saw my personal protection dog, Wendy, lying by my bed cautiously watching everyone who came in. I was shocked and thought for a minute that I was hallucinating, but she *was* there.

"What are you doing here, Wendy? You died two weeks ago?" I asked. She just kept watching the people hustling in and out and replied, "I'm here to watch, just in case." For the first time, I realized that I might not make it.

Finally, the doctor arrived. They put me under and when I awoke a few hours later, the bleeding had stopped and Wendy was gone.

GOD'S HAND AT WORK

As I reflect on that incredible chain of events, I can see clearly how the Hand of God controlled each step. Had the motor home not broken down, I would have been in the middle of nowhere in the San Juaquin Valley, miles from any medical facility, and I would have died. If Dr. Ottaviano had gone to lunch, I would have bled to death with no one to get my heart going again.

With the Master in control, all the circumstances were orchestrated to preserve my life. I didn't know why He would go to all that trouble for common, ordinary me, but I was soon to find out.

What a loving Father we serve. One who never takes His hands off us—not for one minute—even when we are unaware of what He is doing.

That was the last trip I made to California because Dr. Craig passed away and besides, the motor home kept breaking down even more than usual. It had always been a problem to keep repaired, but now when I would fix one thing, two would give out. It got so bad that it was nearly impossible to drive. And since neither the dealer nor the manufacturer would make good on their guarantee, I pasted great big lemon stickers all over it and parked it outside the dealership.

Although my motor-home experience was stressful, it did have its light side, too. On one of my trips home, the bright sun and short sleeping hours made me drowsy. So I pulled over at a closed truck scale to take a nap. That was great, until I heard a bull horn outside my window bellowing, "Hey, what ya' doin' in there? Makin' lemonade?"

When I peeked out the window, a highway patrolman was roaring with laughter as he pulled away. It became the butt of many jokes around dog shows, too. Years later, I met a lady at

Camper World who remembered me from that ridiculous rig. She laughingly informed me that she had a nice new motor home, but had remembered my lemon-mobile and made sure she didn't buy that brand. I didn't get anywhere with the manufacturer or the dealer, but felt justified that I had accomplished something to get revenge.

The closet doors dropped off as we drove. As the wastewater holding tank filled, the weight caused it to fall onto the highway because it was bolted to the floor with only ONE bolt. The radiator overflow tank just fell off one day while I drove down a smooth road. On and on it went.

When I tried to trade the motor home in on another used one, the salesmen laughed me off the lot. After that, I sort of quit trying to drive anywhere in that bomb. The stress was just too much. I never danced a happier jig than I did the day I saw that piece of junk towed out my driveway, even though I did have to buy a new one to unload it.

I wish someone had informed me that depression is a natural reaction to major surgery, or any severe illness, such as a bleeding ulcer like I had experienced. Wendy (the dog that had come to be with me in intensive care), had been quite close to me. She was a trained personal-protection dog that I had bred, raised and trained myself. She took her job very seriously.

The day I finally drove out of Los Angeles, I had Wendy's remains with me so I could bury her at home. As we pulled out of my friends' yard, I felt a thump on the floor of the motor home. Next I felt and heard heavy footsteps trotting down the hall, followed by a jump onto the bed and a heavy thump, as if a large body was deposited there. Out of sheer curiosity, I went back to see and, much to my surprise, half of the bedspread had been bunched up the way Wendy used to "nest" to make it comfortable for herself. The other half had large dog prints indented all over it.

It was quite a shock, but that was the only time I had experienced that. I told her to go on now and enjoy what God had prepared for her, and that I'd see her when I got there. I only saw her one other time after that. I had gotten home around the first of December, but couldn't shake my terrible depression. I was in the backyard cleaning up after the other dogs, feeling sorry for myself as I tearfully talked to God.

"Why didn't you just take me home. Here I am back here trying to make ends meet, too weak to work much, getting sicker and sicker, and all I want to do is sleep and cry." I was having one full-blown pity party until I looked up and saw Wendy running around the outside of the fence, watching me.

I snapped up and asked her, "What are you doing here?" Her answer jolted me out of the doldrums, for she replied, "You have been asking to come, so I came to get you." I dropped to my knees to ask God's forgiveness for despising His gift of life and purpose for me in His scheme of things for the future. When I looked up, she was gone—and so was the depression.

Thank you for using even the death of my beloved dog to bring me back to reality.

I realized that Satan had been trying to kill me, but God had other plans. Those plans began to unfold in February 1990 with the birth of a litter of puppies from my German Shepherd, Beauty. I had waited years for this particular breeding, as it epitomized everything I had been breeding toward. I finally had my line breeding on Phantom, one of the most beautiful, black German Shepherds I'd ever seen. I knew I could get one like him here. (If you've ever been around some of the present-day charismatic circles, you will understand what and why I did next. But if you haven't, you may find it a little strange—as though a lot of what I've related earlier isn't?)

One of those puppies had been born dead. So I put it on a heating pad, cried, fasted and prayed all day for life to come back into this baby. I'd already lost one and I was tenaciously hanging onto this one. I bound Satan, cast him out of my home and away from my animals, and told him to get his hands off these puppies. I belonged to God and so did they. He had no right to them, so get out!

Needless to say, by the end of a long, emotionally draining day, the puppy was still dead. I stood in the kitchen, holding him, while I cried out to God. "Why, Lord, didn't you raise this puppy? You knew how badly I wanted him. And why aren't you healing me? I went forward at The Church On The Way with several thousand people reaching out toward me, packing the place, praying for my healing. John Wimber from The Vinyard was speaking and when he prayed for my healing, he declared that I was healed saying, 'Go in praise to your healer, Jesus Christ of Nazareth.' I did, God, but I've gotten sicker and sicker. And now this? Why aren't you doing anything? You miraculously healed my eyes several years ago and I've seen you heal many, but why not me? I've stood on the Word, I held onto the faith—I did everything I knew. Why?" I sobbed.

His answer came in that same still, quiet voice that has become so distinct and familiar to my inner hearing.

Any disease Satan lays on man, I will remove. And any disease I choose to remove that gives me the glory, I will. But I will not violate my own laws. I made the laws that govern this world and hold it in place. Those laws I will not violate.

Suddenly I saw a vision of a person standing on a railroad track, facing a train that is bearing down on him at top speed.

He is crying out, "Please, God, stop the train. Don't let the train hit me."

He spoke again. *The laws of physics and motion are in effect here. If you don't get off the track, I won't stop the train. If you commit adultery, don't ask me in the middle of it not to let you get pregnant. These are my laws, and I won't stop the sperm from meeting the egg.*

By now, I had quieted down, and meekly asked, "What happened here?" I asked as I looked at the dead puppy.

The law of genetics is what has happened. There was a genetic defect, and I would not violate my law to resurrect this puppy.

"Lord, what should I do? I'm so sick, and everyone believed you'd heal me. What happened in me?" I asked.

There are health laws that have been violated in your body, and in the bodies of thousands just like you, came the response.

"What do I do? How do I get well? You must have saved my life for a purpose, not to just let me die now! That's no glory to you! How can I help anyone else when I can't even heal myself? I'm not a doctor. No one will believe me, and without a medical degree, how can I help anyone, much less myself?" I asked.

His reply was so simple. *You have the greatest physician in the world to teach you, if you will let me. I know what man did to mess this up and I know how to correct it. If you will listen to me and let me guide you, I will teach you what to do. But it will take submission to everything I tell you, and obedience and discipline to get well. If you will agree, someday I will justify you.*

These are my laws. I made them. I will not violate them, and only I know how to correct them. Man too often wants to just sit back and let me do the work of healing him, but doesn't want to suffer the discipline of getting himself well, my way. If they do not listen, they will pay the price.

I was totally awestruck and humbled. As I continued in silence before Him, He reminded me of that time, long ago, when He called me to communicate with animals. I felt the same fear and trembling about stepping out to do something for which others would ridicule me because they didn't understand. Yet He had been true to His word. He did lead me and justify me. Now, as then, I knew I was in for a hard road, but I knew it would be worth it and that He would be there, leading all the way. All I had to do was follow and obey—two seemingly simple words, but oh so dynamic in fulfilling.

"Yes Lord, I don't want to miss out on anything you have for me. I will listen and strive to obey."

Little did I know that I was about to embark on the greatest adventure of my life. There is nothing more exciting than following the Almighty God, being part of His plan as He works His wonders.

Come journey with me into what I believe he has taught me. This is *His* knowledge, *His* work. I am only His hands.

And I love it.

Chapter 7

PIECES OF THE PUZZLE

By late spring, my health had really deteriorated. So I started visiting doctors to see if they had any answers to what I could do about all the tumors on my head, and what caused the tumor that had burst in my stomach.

A biopsy revealed a very rare disease for which there was no known cause or treatment. The disease is called *Sclerosing* (which is a hardening of an organ or tissue due to excessive growth of fibrous tissue, or a thickening and hardening of the layers in the wall of an artery) *Hemangioma* (a benign tumor of dilated blood vessels) *Dermatata* (of the skin) *Fibromata* (a fibrous, encapsulated, connective-tissue tumor, which is slow to grow, irregular in shape, and firm).

I could certainly vouch there were tumors in my stomach because I had seen them when the doctor let me look through the endoscope after the first one had burst. The other one was still there because the doctor didn't want to touch it since it hadn't been bleeding at the time. Several months later, I again noticed bloating and tarry stools, and I began to feel much the way I had when the first one burst the fall before.

This time, instead of a $20,000 hospital bill and a $3,000 doctor bill, I retired to the couch, took yunnan paiyao capsules every couple of hours (they stop internal bleeding) and licorice root (heals the stomach wall), sipped nonacid fruit juice containing psyllium (a bulking agent), and rested. In about a week

I was back to normal, and have never had another problem. This time, treatment cost me only $5.

I continued to use the Herbal Extract to remove the tumors and dissolve them, but they kept growing back. The doctors told me that because the fibrous tumors were lining my blood vessels and my internal organs, a vessel would just close off one day, and I would drop over dead. The physicians could offer no known cause, treatment or hope.

This was a very discouraging time for me because I began to feel that maybe I hadn't heard God right, and I was still going to die. I made out my will, said my good-byes to my family, made preparations for my animals, and waited to die. By then, I was only able to get out of bed about an hour a day. Until one day, that quiet voice spoke to me again and said, *Get out of bed. I'm not finished with you yet.*

Thus began my search for answers through alternative methods of healing.

I knew there had to be something damaged in my body that allowed the tumors to grow back, but didn't know what. So I went back to college to take a refresher course in biology and immunology.

One day, while sitting in class, the teacher was discussing the thymus gland. It was as though a light bulb turned on in my head when he said that this gland, which regulates the rate of growth in the growing child or animal, changes function and configuration in the adult. It then produces T cells, a part of the immune system that literally eats tumors, cancer, tuberculosis, and skin eruptions (cellular diseases).

Since my tumors kept growing back, I knew there had to be a malfunction of my thymus gland, which prevented it from making enough T cells to keep the tumors under control. Allopathic medicine didn't have a clue of what I was looking for, and didn't think I needed to restore the thymus. So I started looking for other ways to restore it.

Many of my alternative-healing friends urged me to use homeopathy, but somehow it didn't ring true with my spirit because homeopathy is basically using the energy of a substance to heal the body. This is a very valid modality for immediate healing since the body is run on energy fields and meridians. But the body also needs living food cells to repair itself. Herbs, God's oldest form of healing, looked like it may hold the answer, so my research began.

About this time, I became aware of others who seemed to be suffering from the same symptoms I was experiencing. Most of them were in the same age range, between 46 and 57. I asked God what this meant and would He please send me an answer? Within a few days, an article arrived in the mail that talked about the Simian 40 virus we got with our polio shot.

I remembered the terrible epidemic that swept the country when we were children. Many of my friends ended up in iron lungs, and we were forbidden to go swimming because the polio virus easily spread through water. In fact, most social functions were canceled to avoid personal contamination.

Everyone was overjoyed when the Salk vaccine was released. Long lines formed in school gyms and health centers so folks could get their shots. But unfortunately, the government couldn't produce enough of it to stop the epidemic.

Now I would like to share with you some excerpts from the article "Retrovirus: The Newcomer," written by Hanna Kroeger (permission for printing is granted by the Hanna Kroeger Foundation):

Here is the story of my life's work. A story so real, so

dramatic, like a fiction, and now thirty years later, thirty years of anguish and suffering, I dare to put this story to paper.

"You cannot go to school unless you are inoculated with the polio vaccine." This was told to my children and many others in the school district of Boulder, Colorado. My children loved school, especially the youngest one, who was in the third grade. She begged me to take her to the place of inoculation. She was proud that she could return to school, the next day.

The third day after her return to school, she had a severe headache and from then on, the school visits became a torture and a total fiasco. Looking back, all of us were in total trust and confidence toward the medical establishment, and we searched our hearts if we the parents were to blame.

The disaster came with unbelievable power, with sicknesses we had never seen before. Not everyone was hit, but I soon found out that the intelligent children of our nation were hit the most.

Soon convulsions set in. Whatever we owned went to the doctor's office, the hospital, and my little girl got worse and worse.

One afternoon, an overworked physician shouted, "If you bring her one more time, we will place her in an institution for the mentally retarded." I felt paralyzed. I sat in the office, my mouth open, all hope was gone. Now I say, "Thank you, physician, you put me on my own two feet."

After this incident, I looked around. I found that other parents became increasingly concerned about their children's behavior. We parents talked it over to compare and to find out what had happened.

It was now summertime. Up in the mountains the so-called "flower children" gathered. They came from everywhere: New York, Los Angeles, San Francisco. And they were from all walks of life. They were doctors' and lawyers' youngsters, they did not groom their hair nor wash their hands. They would injure the business of their parents. "Let them have their own experience and then they will come home" was the slogan at that time. The churches closed the doors against them. The society laughed and made fun of them and they were so sick.

The worst were the nights. I experienced these terrible nights with my own child. Chilled, full of fear, screaming from despair, fever and nausea. For hours, I held my daughter in my arms until she relaxed and slept.

I thought of all the other youngsters. Two youngsters sleeping together in one sleeping bag just to keep warm and offset the fear, the fever, the despair.

The flower children left for warmer climates, but in the coming year, it was worse. One time I asked them not to smoke marijuana because of the danger of destroying the brain stem. The answer was "Can we not feel good and be ourselves once or twice a week?" The smoke helped them to feel better. After that, I never said a single word about marijuana. Is that why marijuana is used? They were sick, as my child was sick, and they got worse month after month. My child had a home, and my child had us, who cared, kept her warm and clean. How about the others in the streets, in the mountains living from rice and bananas.

WHAT HAD HAPPENED

In the end-50s of this century *[I, Beatrice Lydecker, have learned that it happened between the years of about 1949 to 1960]* thousands of little Rhesus apes were shipped to America. They were delivered by the truckloads to laboratories.

With long needles, their little kidneys were pierced and the deadly polio virus was injected. The little animals became deathly ill, the kidneys decomposing with puss and decay.

On the height of their suffering, the Rhesus apes were killed and the puss extracted. This was injected into fertile eggs and after a few days, the famous Salk vaccine was ready to be injected into our children's bloodstream. Many vaccines are made that way; however, here entered the tragedy. The polio virus was dead, but no one knew and no one checked that with this vaccine slipped in a little virus known to be present in apes.

This ape virus has the scientific name of Simian 40, in short, Sim 40. It is a retrovirus, an RNA virus. Sim 40 is harmless to apes, but when entered into the bloodstream of our children, the disaster started.

The big business, the huge propaganda machine, the praise, and the advertisements all subdued the cries of parents whose children were suddenly hit with fear; lack of cleanliness; anguish; failing physical health; failing mental health; depression; laziness; hatred toward parents and teachers; low-grade temperatures; listlessness; and meningitis.

Many more behavioral symptoms were not present before the vaccine was given. Many physicians realized very soon that something went wrong with the inoculations. To avoid more troubles for their patients, they began injecting sterile water until they knew what was going on, and the propaganda machine became occupied with other things.

Sim 40 had never been in human blood before, and all at once, millions of Americans had it. Sim 40 ... an RNA virus found in apes, sheep, cattle and mice. It is a virus that can change according to the environment it is bathed in, and also the amount of life energy or lack of life it gets. ...

Many [people with this virus] have seen the horror of mental institutions. Many committed suicide. Many have seen jails from inside, and many just existed. ...

According to medical textbooks and also veterinarian textbooks and also research done at C.U., Sim 40 is an RNA virus [that] goes into the nervous system. It hides in the spinal fluid, in the nervous system, and [those infected] feel tension in the back of their necks and between their shoulder blades

Of all the viruses, the retrovirus is the most feared ... because it can stay dormant for many, many years. It will strike whenever the system becomes low in energy.

In spite of all our doings, our daughter got worse and worse. She was 15 now. She had been diagnosed with lympho sarcoma, lympho leukemia, hepatitis C, swollen belly, and blindness. Death was close.

I called Dr. Burwell and asked her what I should do. She answered, and it was the right answer, "Let her go, she suffered so much." So, I was sitting at her bedside, holding her little white hand in mine. I had placed a red rose on her chest so she could leave more easily, and I whispered the childhood verses she knew.

She then stretched and she was gone.

I closed my eyes and said the Lord's prayer. I came to the end and looked at her white sunken face. There it was, a tear, first in her right eye, then in her left. I moistened her dry lips with a cotton sponge and waited. She moved one finger, then one hand. She then opened her mouth and wanted to say something. I waited and prayed. All of a sudden, she asked, "Mother, what is a mission?"

"A mission," I said, "is a promise to God to do something for Him."

Somewhat later she told me. "I was in a beautiful place, lavender, blue and white. Many people were standing or sitting, and whoever raised their hand was lifted up to Jesus, who was in front. It was so peaceful and I lifted up my hand, but a voice said, 'You have not fulfilled your mission, go back.'" She cried," I want to go there—to the light. I belong there."

"Honey, let us fulfill this mission together," I said. "Let us work hard. Our Lord spoke to you that is holy to both of us."

Weeks of despair, weeks of suicide tendencies. We couldn't leave her alone. She stabbed herself with dull kitchen knives. She went to the lake to drown herself. "I don't want to stay alive, I want to go to the light," was her daily prayer.

Looking back, it was a nightmare, a total nightmare. Weeks went by and she gained strength. Her seizures became less frequent. Her eyesight returned, her hearing improved. My daily prayer was "Oh Lord, please show me the mission which we have to fulfill." And He, Our Lord, did show us. It was a battle of thirty years to find the truth, to find the answer. Bits and pieces of knowledge filtered through.

The terrible times of flower children and suicidal youngsters was over. Many young people never went back to school. They could not think. They could only do manual labor for four to five hours and, exhausted, they lay on their cots for hours and hours. When they overworked, fever and chills set in. No appetite, no strength. The youth and people of our time are the carriers of this terrible virus.

The retrovirus, an animal virus, not recognized, not understood, and not an ounce of medication to help.

PIECES OF THE PUZZLE

SCIENCE SPEAKS

I had the unbelievable good luck to meet a lady physician from Switzerland. She visited Boulder to find out why America's youth behaved so strangely ("Flower Children," "Hippie Children"). I told her the story of my child and the many other sick children without help and without hope. I told her that it came after the Rhesus apes were used for carriers of vaccination.

She listened quietly. Then she jumped up, took me by my shoulders and shook me. "Tell this once more," she said, "Please!" I said it again and then she answered: "I was in Lambarene with Dr. Albert Schweitzer. I was there for three months. When someone came for help to the clinic that had been bitten by an ape, Dr. Schweitzer did not help. He was standing in the doorway crying because he had to send them back into the jungles to die. He explained: 'Apes have a very potent virus. When this virus goes into the bloodstream of a human being through the bite of a monkey or other infected animal, or an infected needle, this virus settles into the nervous system. It is contagious and there is no help known. There will come a time when we can help, but not now.'"

These monkey viruses have also been deadly in the laboratory. Here is ... a quote from Dr. Gallo: "Marburg virus belongs to a new class of RNA viruses. It was discovered in 1967 after an outbreak in Europe in which thirty-one people were infected and seven died. It began when a virus from African green monkeys infected laboratory scientists who were working with the monkey's kidneys."

The following information is taken from the books *The Human Retrovirus* and *Virus Hunting* by Robert C. Gallo, M.D. Dr. Gallo writes: "Retroviruses are originally found in animals. An animal can live with the retrovirus. This does not hurt them. Mice, apes and sheep are known to carry this virus. When mutton is cooked and eaten, the meat cannot hurt you because it enters the stomach and the digestive tract, which is full of enzymes that kill the virus. However, if sheep serum or ape serums are used for making an antidote for different diseases, we have a different story."

I would like to interject my concern about attention-deficit disorder (ADD). It has long been my belief that it is caused by a virus or something contained in the diphtheria or whooping-cough vaccinations. I have seen many of my clients whose children were normal yet developed this problem on the heels of the diphtheria shot.

Even Dr. Dean Adel commented on his radio show that the vaccine was defective (he had been talking about the affects it had on a listener's son who had been normal until the day after he received the vaccination).

ADD affects mostly males, attacking their nervous systems. I believe it affects females differently and is behind scleroderma, which you will notice affects mostly females and has no known etiology or cause. And how about the former Miss America who went deaf after a diphtheria shot, but later had to change her story to say they didn't know why she had gone deaf? Also, did you know that the dyphtheria shot is made by using sheep's blood, and is preserved with mercury and aluminum? Although I can't prove it, this seems very dangerous in light of what Gallo revealed about sheep's blood carrying a retrovirus.

It was not known that apes carry such a deadly virus until the tragedy in the end of the 1950s. At this time, millions of Americans received the retrovirus Simian 40 directly into their bloodstream through the polio vaccine. (Inoculations were given over a period of about eleven years, but when scientists learned that the vaccination carried the retrovirus, they switched back to growing the Salk vaccine on yeast and giving it on a sugar cube. So the vaccine became safe since it no longer involved apes. Sad to say, this knowledge came too late. The damage had been done and millions of Americans—most of the baby-boomers—are now infected.

Now let's get back to Hanna's story:

I present now documentation [from the files of the National Health Institute in Bethesda, Maryland] about retroviruses. A quote from Dr. Gallo: "Only once in its early history did the Institute take a seriously false step. In 1954, during the height of the polio epidemic, the March of Dimes foundation 'ordered five drug companies to begin producing mass lots of (polio) vaccine, on the basis of a formula for inactivating the virus with formaldehyde,' according to a procedure the polio researcher Jonas Salk himself has devised."

Samples of the inactivated vaccine were then sent to the N.I.H. Laboratory of Biologic Control, which was responsible for certifying that the vaccines were indeed inactivated and safe for use. The actual testing was done by Dr. Bernice Eddy. Using eighteen monkeys as test animals, Eddy and her staff began inoculating the animals with a vaccine from each of the five drug companies. With one particular sample, the test monkeys showed signs of paralysis, an indication that these lots of vaccine had not been properly inactivated. Although she reported her findings to the appropriate authorities at N.I.H., she heard nothing more about it. In fact, one of her superiors asked her whether she should like to have her own children inoculated, since there was not enough vaccine for every child in America. Not surprisingly, Eddy demurred.

Eddy [is quoted as saying],"They went ahead and released the vaccine anyway, a lot of it. The monkeys they just disregarded." The only surprising thing was that the consequences weren't even more horrible than they actually were. Eighty children received active vaccine. Now harboring active virus, presumably through inoculation, they passed it on to approximately one hundred and twenty additional people with whom they came in contact. By the time the error was discovered, three-quarters of the victims had been paralyzed and eleven had died. A national furor followed. By the time it ended, the director of microbiology institute had lost his post, and both the secretary of Health Education and Welfare and the director of the N.I.H. had resigned.

For more information, read some of the following books:
Beneson, A., *Control of Communicable Diseases in Man.* American Public Health Associations, 1985.

Gallo, R., *Virus Hunting.* A New Republic Book Basic Books, 1991.

Gallo, R., and Gilbert, J., *The Human Retroviruses.* Academic Press, 1991.

Koneman, E., et al. *Diagnostic Microbiology.* Third edition. J.B. Lippincott Co., 1988.

When I read the article by Hanna Kroeger, I thanked God for her courage to stand up and voice the truth so seldom heard in today's medically oriented, self-protecting society. I can also understand why the N.I.H. and the government don't want this information widely known, for every sufferer may want to start a lawsuit.

That also explains why they went on such a campaign to discredit Gallo and make him look so bad that people wouldn't listen to him or take him seriously. They did a good job with their smear tactics. The government is really good at that. I must say one thing in their defense, though: I don't believe they deliberately started out to infect society. I believe that they honestly made a mistake (or at least my Americanism wants to believe it) in using monkeys to grow the polio vaccine. Unfortunately, in their haste to get the Salk vaccine produced in mass—enough to stop the epidemic—they made some horrible mistakes by not checking out what may come along with it.

Although the situation was tragic, I was relieved to discover all these things. I remembered what God had spoken to me—that He knew what man had done to mess things up and here it was. In faithfulness to His prophetic word to me, He had brought it to my attention. Now that He had, I began to pray for a deeper understanding of this virus and what it does to the body and how to correct it, as He had promised He would teach me.

This was turning into a VERY exciting adventure.

Over the next few months, the following information came into my hands through various sources. As bits and pieces came in, it all began to fit together like pieces of a puzzle. This is the final picture that emerged.

All Retroviruses Lack DNA

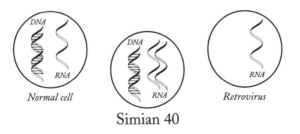

Normal cell

Simian 40

Retrovirus

WHAT'S A VIRUS AND HOW'S THIS ONE DIFFERENT FROM THE OTHERS

In every cell there are two codes: DNA and RNA. The DNA is the genetic code that tells you what you will look like. If your parents are black, you will be black. If your parents are blond-haired and blue-eyed, you probably will be, too. These are the genes that you inherit from your ancestors.

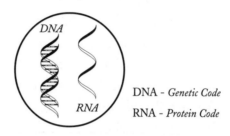

DNA - *Genetic Code*
RNA - *Protein Code*

The second is the RNA, a protein code that determines the makeup of your cell wall, the protein part of your body.

Now, in order for a virus to work in your body, it must invade your cells and use your cells to survive. Antibiotics do not kill viruses. They only kill organisms such as bacteria and protozoa that float around in your bloodstream, and the virus is *hidden* in the cells of your body. In most cases, the body can produce antibodies that can kill the virus wherever it is hiding. It may take a few days to do, so a cold virus will usually run its course in about ten days.

Supporting the body with vitamin C and fluids will help the body defend itself faster, but there are very few actual virus-killer substances on the market (the Herbal Extract usually can knock out the average virus in about four days).

The Simian 40 virus is very different. It invades the cell, bonds with the RNA in that cell, and TRICKS that cell into thinking it is the Simian 40 virus—making that cell a manu-

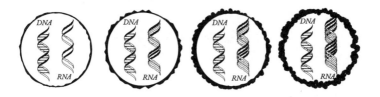

facturing plant for the virus. The body may build some antibodies toward it, but because it uses the cell to gain strength and replicate itself, the body cannot kill it off. At the time of this writing, I personally only know of one thing that can eventually kill it: Living Free Herbal Extract. But it takes time.

Every cell of our body has a very porous wall, which allows oxygen and nutrients to get into the cell to rebuild it and give it nourishment to function. When nutrients are burned, the byproduct is waste that needs to be eliminated from the cell, the same way ashes need to be removed from a stove to allow room for oxygen and new fuel to have a place to burn. When the Simian 40 virus enters the cell and bonds with the RNA, the virus changes the configuration of the cell wall and gradually plugs the pores, thus blocking the cell's ability to get oxygen and nutrients and clean out the waste. The process is very slow, sometimes taking years, making it appear as though the virus is lying dormant when it is not.

I can see no way science could *ever* kill it because it is a retrovirus, which means that it changes the configuration of the cell walls every time it spreads to a different host. By the time they discover how to kill one configuration, it has spread through many new hosts, changing again and again and again.

Therefore, we must have a way to kill it in whatever form we find it, in whatever host it is living. I believe we have done that. I'll explain how in the next chapter.

A LIST OF DISEASES THAT RESULT FROM THE *SIMIAN 40* RETROVIRUS

1. HIV
2. Fibromyalgia
3. Epstein-Barr Virus
4. Hepatitis C
5. MS
6. Lupus
7. Chronic Fatigue Syndrome
8. Non-Hodgkin's Lymphoma
9. Post-Polio Syndrome

WHY SIMIAN 40 IS CALLED BY DIFFERENT NAMES

Science tends to look at symptoms and name a disease by the symptoms it produces. This virus seems to be the common thread running through multiple diseases, but because of where it expresses itself, science thinks they are different. I believe in reality that they have the same root cause: Simian 40.

These diseases are called by the following names:

- Lenti virus (an ape virus): becomes a retrovirus in humans.
- Simian 40 (an ape virus): becomes a retrovirus in humans.
- HIV I and II: attacks the cells of the thymus gland and matured T cells.
- Hepatitius C (non-A, non-B): attacks the cells of the liver.
- Adult T-cell leukemia: attacks the immature T cells in the bone.
- Non-Hodgkin's lymphona.
- Chronic Fatigue, CFIDS, Fibromyalgia, Epstein-Barr: attacks the cells of muscle tissue.

In combination with other viruses and fungi, the retrovirus can also be found in the following:

- Lymph cell sarcoma: attacks the lymphocyte or white blood cells in the lymph glands.
- T-cell lymphoma sarcoma: attacks the matured T cells in the lymph glands, making it appear like it is a cancer of the T cells.
- Peripheral T-cell lymphoma: attacks the T cells of the extremities.
- Lupus: attacks the cells of the skin and connective tissue causing chronic inflammation of the connective tissues.
- Multiple sclerosis: attacks the cells of the connective tissue and the myelon sheath in the spinal cord.
- Hairy cell leukemia: attacks the blood cells and tissue of the spleen, often causing anemia by decomposition of the blood cells.

In addition to the above, Dr. Neiper from Germany stated that a retrovirus is very frequently found in breast cancer also.

When we look at all these diseases that have the same root virus, we have found that when we approach them all with the same four-step program, we get the same results: the person gets well! In fact, when I work with *any* major disease using the Four-Step Program, I've found it's important to clean the body systems and rebuild them. When we do, the body can fight off most diseases.

GULF WAR SYNDROME AND BIOLOGICAL WARFARE

The biological agents used in warfare, such as in the Gulf War, attack the cells of the body indiscriminately, bond with the DNA, which is the genetic code of the cell, and alter it. This includes the reproductive cells. Thus, 66 percent of the Gulf War veterans who took the pesticide pill (which destroys the immune system, giving the biological opportunity to do its work) produced offspring with birth defects, according to Maj. Joyce Riley, who has done extensive work with the Gulf War veterans.

The Four-Step Program has been effective in helping these victims, particularly those who contacted it from an infected individual. When one is first infected, the best treatment is with Doxycycline or its sister drug, Tetracycline. But once it has taken hold, the drugs only seem to hold some of the symptoms. I'll explain what to do in more detail in a later chapter that describes various illnesses.

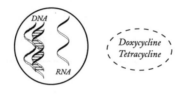

Gulf War Syndrome

SECTION II

Healing the Body

*My people are destroyed
for lack of knowledge.*

HOSEA 4:6

«FOUR-STEP»
PROGRAM

---

1. Clean & Restore
   the Liver

2. Kill Parasites

3. Clean & Restore
   the Immune System

4. Kill Viruses & Tumors

Chapter 8

KEYS TO HEALTH:
The Four-Step Program

I now had the "What," and how it got into the population. What was the next step? I needed to fully understand how the body systems work, and how this virus affected it in order to know how to correct it. That information was soon to be put into my hands, too. As that knowledge increased, the Four-Step Program gradually took shape.

STEP ONE

One day I received a booklet in the mail explaining all about the liver, the processing plant of our body. It made me aware that rebuilding the liver is the first key to restoring and maintaining health. It makes no difference what you eat, if the liver is not healthy and functioning at full capacity, you cannot process food, and you will never get well.

Chronic constipation is one of the main signs that the liver is congested. Another sign is the presence of liver spots on the hands, arms and face. When you clean and rebuild the liver, spots fade and constipation ceases.

What Does This Incredible Organ Do?

There is so much to be said about it that I could do a whole book on just this organ alone. But I will limit the information to only the bare essentials you'll need to know to restore it.

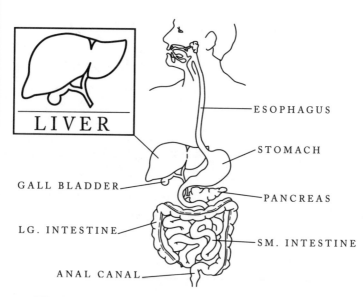

ESOPHAGUS

STOMACH

GALL BLADDER

PANCREAS

LG. INTESTINE

SM. INTESTINE

ANAL CANAL

Digestive System (esp. Liver)

1. Manufactures bile and stores it in gall bladder.

2. Liver produces 13,000 chemicals. Donor match: Must match like fingerprint.

3. Liver produces 2,000 Enzymes (+).

4. Repairs Heart: Converts CoQ_{1-9} into CoQ_{10} and sends it to the heart.

5. Produces ortho-phospho tyrosine, a growth hormone.

When you eat food, it passes through the mouth where lipase works on the carbohydrates you eat. It then passes to the stomach, where the hydrochloric acid is produced, which is vital to breakdown the proteins and calcium into molecules small enough for the body to utilize.

If you take an antacid with your meals, you destroy the stomach's ability to perform this function. The calcium then gets into the bloodstream in whole molecules where it could stick to the good cholesterol on the blood vessel walls and possibly result in arteriosclerosis. If the protein isn't broken down in the stomach, it will pass into the small intestines where, since it also is in molecules too large to be absorbed, it will ferment and cause gas, eventually passing through the body, mostly unused.

In many individuals, there is already an inherited deficiency of hydrochloric acid, making them very "gassy" whenever they eat protein. These individuals, along with those who are hypothyroid, can also become calcium deficient since they are unable to utilize what they have consumed. Taking HCL with each meal will help alleviate this problem, but I don't recommend it. If you take enzymes, you will always be dependent on them.

You should instead stimulate the body's natural ability to do the job it was designed to do. Once it is functioning properly, you'll be able to get off all supplementation. The Digestion Formula seems to do that while it also stops acid reflux, naturally.

Correct the Problem. Don't Spend the Rest of Your Life Controlling Symptoms

As the food passes into the duodenum or small intestine, the pancreas secretes insulin to metabolize the sugars. The gallbladder, which is only a storage bag for bile manufactured in the liver, also dumps into the duodenum several times a day, releasing bile to emulsify any fats it finds there.

If you have had your gallbladder removed, then the fat cannot be emulsified until it reaches the liver, making that organ work harder than it should. When you eat fats in the absence of a gallbladder, drink oolong tea, eat flax seed, use flax seed oil (great mixed with butter to cut the fat and add flavor), or take lecithin to emulsify the fat before it reaches the liver.

I once did a test on one of my obese German Shepherds and found that 50 percent of her blood was fat. So I put her on one lecithin capsule of 1,200 mg per day, and in just thirty days, the fat was gone from her bloodstream!

Once the food is sufficiently broken down in the small intestine, it is absorbed through the walls, into the bloodstream, where it is carried to the liver for processing.

The liver produces about 2,000 enzymes and thousands of synergists to enable the body to convert the foods you eat into living cells that match your body cells. The lettuce, fruit, meat and so on are composed of a different type of cell from yours and must be converted in the liver so it will match your cell structure. Once the cells are "humanized," they are sent, via the bloodstream, to the tissues to repair them.

You can help this process even further by adding four herbs—cinnamon, clove, red root and Irish moss—to the diet, as they are pro-enzymes, which makes much less work by the liver.

The nutrients that the liver has extracted from the food is now sent to the tissue cells to nourish them. An example of this is the processing of the CoQ enzymes. It amazes me how the liver can realize when the heart needs CoQ_{10} to repair it. The liver takes the CoQ enzymes 1 through 9 from the foods you eat (such as organ meats, mackerel, sardines, eggs, broccoli, potatoes, spinach, rice, wheat, corn, pistachio nuts, walnuts, peanuts, chestnuts, almonds and sesame seeds), converts them to CoQ_{10}, and sends it to the heart to repair it.

When one has a heart condition, one usually already has a weakened or problem liver that can't convert the CoQ enzymes or even extract them from foods. This makes it important to not only treat the heart, but makes a lot of sense to treat the liver first. If you don't, you are treating symptoms and not the root problem. Even if you take CoQ_{10} as a supplement, unless the liver is functioning at full capacity, even the supplement will pass through, unused.

One thing we do find in holistic or natural healing is the phenomenon that "like organs repair like organs." Because the tissue is similar in mammals, if you have a weakened liver, we recommend eating liver; if you have a diseased kidney, take kidney in some form, and so on. The liver is somehow able to recognize the similarity between your organ and the other mammal's organ, and sends those cells to the proper organ to repair it. I have had many vegetarians contact me to ask for my products free of glandulars (which are extracted from beef or sheep). I'm sorry, but I just haven't found the formulas to work anywhere near as effectively, so I can't do it.

Once the nutrients have been burned by the cells, the cell waste is then carried by the bloodstream to the liver and spleen, and by the lymph glands to the kidneys where these systems are "cleaned." The waste is then deposited into the large intestine or colon through a hepatic shunt or duct, where it is carried out of the body.

If the liver doesn't work efficiently, then it can't clean the blood, but leaves the toxins or waste there to be deposited in the joints and fatty tissue or is sent to the kidneys, stressing those organs as they try to eliminate it. This often occurs when you are killing parasites, diseased tissues, and so on. It overloads the liver and spleen, so the kidneys have to pick up the extra process. The liver, spleen and kidneys all working together are greatly taxed in the elimination of toxins or dead tissue and, if not properly supported, could get congested or shut down. This is especially true when the patient suffers from hepatitis, cirrhosis or cancer of the liver. That is the reason we include a small bottle of Kidney Support Formula with the program, as it only takes a few days to relieve the kidney pain and get them back to full capacity.

Joint pain can easily be confused with arthritis, when in reality, it could be toxicity. As the liver is repaired, often the "arthritis" vanishes. I have had several clients say they were diagnosed as having arthritis, but when they had their mercury fillings replaced with the mercury-free plastics or porcelain, the "arthritis" mysteriously disappeared. When you are toxic from either mercury or have overloaded the liver, you will often feel tired, sluggish, achy and unable to think clearly. You can usually quickly alleviate those symptoms by flushing the body with lots of extra water and apple juice and by taking two natural detoxifiers, charcoal and alpha lipoic acid.

I cannot emphasize enough how vital it is to the patient's survival and complete recovery from any major illness to do ongoing liver cleanses and stimulation to rebuild it.

It is VERY IMPORTANT to watch what you think, especially when trying to restore these three organs. Feelings of anger, defeatism, fear, self-pity and resentment make the liver produce chemicals that slow down the repair processes of the body, creating an adverse acidic condition.

Now I know what God meant when He said in Proverbs 17:22, "A merry heart does good, like medicine." That's why I put that verse on all my checks.

The liver produces 13,000 chemicals that make you distinctly you. I always marvel at the incredible ability dogs have to identify people by being able to distinguish the slightest difference in their chemical makeup. When doctors are trying to make a match for donor organs, they are attempting to match more than blood type. They are trying to match as closely as possible the chemicals. Since there are no perfect matches, they must suppress the immune system, or it will attempt to destroy the foreign object.

Again, the liver functions as an incredible instrument. It produces a growth hormone called ortho-phospho tyrosine. When the liver identifies a foreign body of any kind is present, whether it be a donated organ, a sliver or a parasite, it sends the growth hormone to the cells around the object, making them grow rapidly or "out of control," encasing or killing the object.

If you have ever had the opportunity to see a liver infected by liver flukes, you will see the parasite encased in a callused, pus-filled sac, which is the body's attempt to isolate the culprit. I believe this is how benign or malignant tumors grow. The liver is attempting to isolate a parasite. Unfortunately, the parasite also gets the growth hormone and as it continues to grow along with the cells surrounding it, the tumor gets larger and larger.

Isn't this what a cancerous tumor really is, a localized group of cells growing out of control? To control tumor growth, wouldn't it make more sense to kill the parasite or suppress the growth hormone rather than to destroy the immune system when you are already dealing with an immune-compromised disease?

Chemo only helps reduce or control the cancer less than 35 percent of the time. And radiation causes another form of inflammatory or tissue cancer later on. What do you think came out of Three Mile Isle in Pennsylvania and Chernobyl in

Russia? Why do you think there is so much controversy over nuclear plants? It's radiation from these that caused so much cancer around them.

One more warning about chemo: Doctors will never tell you that, since chemo is a poison, it can cause an allergic reaction in the lungs. The lungs may fill up with fluid and drown you, but doctors will say you have "developed pneumonia." DON'T LET THEM FOOL YOU.

A very sweet mother in her early 40s (with a vulnerable teenage daughter) came to me with lympho sarcoma. Sandy, who lived in Vancouver, Washington, had developed breast cancer, and after her mastectomy, the cancer spread to the lymph glands. When I first saw her, she had been undergoing chemo for FIVE YEARS. Unbelievable! If it hadn't worked in a short time, but allowed the cancer to spread, why would anyone in his or her right mind—even the doctors—continue the same unsuccessful treatment? Could it have been for the money?

During her last several treatments, Sandy began to experience a buildup of fluid in her lungs, but the kicker came with the last one she had before I met her. The fluid had become so severe (and happened within minutes of injecting the chemo) that they needed to insert a needle directly into the lungs and draw out the fluid to keep her from drowning.

When I first saw her, her neck looked as though she had a huge cauliflower inserted under the skin, the tumors were huge and profuse, and she was bedridden and constantly on oxygen. She couldn't even eat anymore, for even a grape filled her up.

I didn't know much of what I do now, but we did start her on the Herbal Extract. Three weeks later, she was off the oxygen, her neck was back to normal and she was out of bed—even able to walk when someone helped her to her feet. She was able to eat and had even gained a few pounds.

We were thrilled, only to experience a tremendous heart-break a week later. Her doctors called her and told her to come back for another chemo treatment. We urged her not to, to just give the herbs a chance. But as doctors usually do, they used scare tactics and intimidation to get her to come back. Their tactics usually work with people so sick that their weakened condition makes them emotionally very vulnerable.

Her doctors were trying to say that their chemo treatments were finally working. (After *five* years? Give me a break!) And if she didn't keep it up, she would die.

Much to everyone's despair, the chemo treatment killed her. As they injected the chemo, her lungs immediately filled with fluid and no effort on their part could clear them this time, and she drowned.

This was not the first or last time we have had this happen to one of our clients. One of them lived in Bakersfield, California. She came to us because the chemo hadn't worked. She stopped the treatments and went on the Herbal Extract. Several months later, she was declared by her doctor to be clear of cancer, all traces of it gone. But they intimidated her into going for one more chemo treatment "just to be sure we got it all" (as though they thought they had succeeded).

When she went in for the treatment, they overdosed her and she drowned. I am relating just these two cases, but could give you case after case of the same thing happening to others we know or have helped—only to have doctors and hospitals kill them.

How can they call it "developing pneumonia" when it happens within minutes of a chemo injection? Since when does pneumonia happen that fast? When I heard on the news that Jackie Kennedy Onassis, who was undergoing chemo for cancer, had developed "pneumonia," I knew her days were going to be very short. I knew they were drowning her and, sure enough, she died within days of the announcement.

If you ever hear that I have "committed suicide" or come up missing, don't believe a word of it. I have too much faith in God to do anything like that. I've been through too much to give up now. The medical profession has a way of burying their mistakes and charging you for it. They also have a way of burying those who expose their little games or help people get well. Every one of them ends up dead, their records missing, their reputations smeared—or they themselves just "disappear" if they don't want to end up in jail.

Those closest to me have asked that I not tell the full truth because they fear for me. But I would be remiss and unfaithful to God if I didn't tell you the whole truth. Then and only then can you protect yourself and your family. (The closest science has ever come to doing it right is using the chemo drug called Toxol, a sheep dewormer.)

The medical profession has seen the writing on the wall. So they have, in some states such as California, passed laws making it illegal to treat cancer with anything other than chemo and radiation. They have even gone so far as to take people's children away from them—and do it themselves—if a parent wishes to use any other treatment.

I know, for one day I was called by a mutual acquaintance who was trying to help a mother find a safe hiding place where she could treat her child with alternatives for his cancer. The authorities were coming to take him to a hospital and force chemo and radiation on him.

They know that people who have become aware of the low survival rate of those submitted to doctors' methods are turning to alternatives in larger and larger numbers.

The doctors and hospitals are the only ones benefiting from the tremendously high costs involved in these treatments. They don't want to lose the hundreds of thousands of dollars it is costing the poor patients and their families (to say nothing of the human suffering they are causing). So they have taken this measure to protect their industry.

I am asked almost daily if our program will work along with chemo and radiation. Yes, it will, but you will take three steps forward and two backward. You will eventually get there, but it will take you longer.

Should cancer strike the liver or the lungs, you have to go very slowly in killing it. These are highly vascular systems and if you go too fast, you could take a blood vessel wall with the cancer as you kill it. The body has to have time to rebuild healthy tissue as it kills off the bad.

I cannot overemphasize the importance of heavily oxygenating the body when cancer strikes these two organs. Oxygen kills disease and nowhere is it more needed than in these organs. You can use stabilized oxygen in water, but do not add it to acidic juices like orange juice. The acid will break the sodium bond and release the oxygen in the juice, instead of in your stomach, where the hydrochloric acid needs to release it, making it more accessible to the bloodstream directly through the stomach wall. An Ozonator machine is another wonderful source of "pure," more concentrated oxygen. Or just try breathing pure oxygen with a mask or a nasal cannula hooked to an oxygen tank.

One other strange phenomenon concerning the liver: It will cause the body to crave what it is allergic to. For example, if a person is allergic to sugar, they will have an uncontrollable craving for sweets, similar to the way the hypoglycemic craves carbohydrates and sugar. As the liver becomes healthy, the cravings decrease. But if the cravings do not subside, one needs to examine his or her emotional issues (for example, a poor person will crave the staples of life such as pasta and potatoes, while a person who feels they are missing out on the good, "sweet" things in life will crave sweets).

There are three things you can do to help control those cravings. First, you can use alpha lipoic acid and the solution VanChroZin (vanadium, chromium and zinc), both of which regulate blood sugar levels, thus cutting the cravings.

Second, the more sweets you eat, the worse it gets, so you have to go cold turkey and break the metabolic cycle. This can be done by "fasting" sweets for three days. It breaks the metabolism and helps stop the hold the cravings have on you. It is like an alcoholic. You can't even take a little or you'll go right back to it. By the way, alcohol and sugar break down in the bloodstream to exactly the same molecules. So when you stop drinking, you will greatly crave sweets or vice versa. Heavy sugar intake can also damage the liver as alcoholism does; it just takes a little longer for the damage to show up.

Third, the liver will also cause cravings if there is a deficiency of molybdenum. So you may want to get that checked.

In the light of all this information, I realized that for the first five days we need to start cleaning the liver and make it function at full capacity. Then, whatever else we do or consume will be effectively processed and clean the blood completely. This is accomplished by starting with the Liver/Gall Bladder Formula. Wouldn't it be better to restore your own liver than to look for an expensive transplant that requires a suppression of your immune system for the rest of your life? This only leaves you open to the possibility of succumbing to another disease because you have lost your immune defenses.

I was amazed to learn that the liver is the only organ that can regrow when a section is removed. Wow! God made sure that crucial organ was renewable! When I understood how incredibly just this one organ of the body works, I stood in awe at God who created it so perfectly. Truly, "we are fearfully and wonderfully made."

STEP TWO

In all my research and experience, I have found that everyone who has any major illness has a weakened immune system resulting in the inability to throw off parasites. This could be worms, bacterium, or a protozoa such as cryptospyridium, which is commonly found in the drinking water of large cities. It causes severe diarrhea in immune-suppressed individuals like AIDS and cancer victims. It cannot be killed by chlorine, but can with oxygen.

This is done by installing an Ozonator machine in your drinking-water system, like Los Angeles did a few years ago before the Olympics. It works by turning O_2 into O_3, a more concentrated form of oxygen that kills many pathogens. O_2 is commonly found in our air. It rises, penetrating the ozone layer to reach the sun, where it is converted into O_3. It then drops back down to earth to sterilize the air. You can recognize it by that wonderful fragrance present after a fresh rain.

I have an Ozonator and I love it. It removes the bacteria in the air that causes odors, purifies the water, and supplies better oxygen for breathing. Some of my clients also use it to purify their swimming pools and hot tubs instead of the toxic chlorine.

The second step in getting well is to rid the body of parasites so that everything taken in will be used by the body and not by the parasites. On day six we add Copper Solution, which kills all kinds of parasites, including tapeworms. I can hear many of you saying, "I don't have parasites. I don't live in a third-world country."

Well, in my experience I have found that everyone with any major disease is immune suppressed and has parasites. The most common ones are flukes of all kinds and pinworms (also called threadworms). If you experience itching in your ears, nose, around your eyes or rectum (especially at night), it is probably pinworms. These two are easily eliminated. Why do we think children get them so easily and we as adults won't?

Where is contamination coming from? FOOD! Parasite eggs are microscopic so you can't see them. Most of our foods are picked by migrant workers from contaminated, third-world countries. With no bathrooms in the fields or orchards, workers have no place to wash their hands. And since farmers don't require them to show proof of deworming, contamination is spread.

Simply washing with plain water doesn't kill contamination. You have to use oxygen or chlorine baths. How about food handlers in restaurants and grocery stores? Have you ever taken a cruise where nearly all the crew is from the Philippines and other tropical islands where sanitation is practically nonexistent? I have been on several, and every time I come home, I have brought a few "passengers" with me (including viruses from the closed-filter systems). I always deworm when I come back from a trip like that, and I always find them.

If you have ever handled a lot of animals, you probably have them, too. I used to do acupuncture on my friend's bulls and, believe me, there is nothing except pigs that are dirtier. I am still fighting a tapeworm in my sinus that comes from dogs. (I have seen the segments, even though I am told you can't get them from dogs.) Thank God for the copper water (made from the natural element found in trace minerals, not the dangerous stuff from pipes) because it is now dying. My sinuses are clearing up and my hearing is getting better.

But would I give up my beloved animals? Not on your life! They give me so much more that is positive, it far outweighs my need to take a little Copper Solution once in awhile. They are well worth it! Besides, I travel a lot and need to deworm regularly anyway. If we don't start addressing them in the adult population, we will soon reach epidemic proportions—in fact, I think we already have!

Sometimes it is hard to find them by stool samples. I've had several tests done, but the laboratory kept telling me I didn't have any. I decided to treat myself anyway and started with wormword, black walnut tincture and cloves (to kill the eggs that parasites give off as they die).

For several weeks, I saw flukes in every stage of development, but still felt I had more. One of the major symptoms of tapeworms is the bloated feeling I experienced every time I ate, even small amounts. So I decided to use the herb called rascal. It contains cayenne pepper, which is supposed to kill them. But all I got was heartburn, no parasites. Finally I got desperate and decided to take a strong drug called Praziquantel or Biltricide, commonly called Droncit for dogs, which cost $140 through the local pharmacy. During my next trip to Mexico, I purchased the same thing, made by the same pharmaceutical company, for less than $40.

For more than a year, I had been experiencing a steady ache in my descending colon, but when I took the Praziquantel, it stopped and has never come back. Previously I had seen what looked like mucous on my stools, only to learn they were segments of fish tapeworms (all fish are loaded with tapeworms as well as mercury). When I finally killed it, it was so large it took a week to pass the whole thing. It had to have been several feet long in my intestines, yet I had been told repeatedly that I didn't have any parasites. Another thing I passed were large balls of beef tapeworms, wound around each other like the insides of a baseball. They are dark brown and segmented, about three to five inches long, clumped together in what are called "nests."

I have met several people who experience pain in their upper arms and shoulders when they try to lift their arms above their heads. I had visited with several doctors and chiropractors, but none of them could find an answer or help at all. Finally, because I was also experiencing tremendous itching just above the elbow, I decided to try painting it with the Herbal Extract. The more I applied, the worse it itched until it gradually opened up, leaving gaping holes (which didn't bleed) in my arm. Much to my surprise, when I was finally able to look into the holes, I was shocked to see long, white worms embedded in the muscle tissue. When I looked them up in a book on parasites, I discovered they were trichinella.

The symptoms of trichinosis matched so much of what I was experiencing, they were masked until the parasites had finally imbedded themselves in the muscles of my arms. I then took Thiabendazole for twenty days, but on day 15, the itching and pain became almost unbearable. I stuck it out and went on with the treatment. Within a few hours it had stopped, and so had the itching and the pain, even when I lifted my arm high above my head.

Taking all that medicine, including several weeks of Mebendazol, Albendazol, and Biltricide, really affected my liver. I know it did because the brown spots on the back of my hands got larger and darker. Once it was over and I continued to clean my liver with the Liver Formula, they gradually faded. Most disappeared, and those that didn't, got much smaller (a common reaction observed in many of our clients). This was a hard program to follow because we were swallowing so many pills each day, some of which I knew were hard on the liver we were trying to help. Remember, they are called liver spots for a reason.

I am so thankful I finally discovered the Copper Solution, which even kills tapeworms. It is cheaper and easier to take (only a couple tablespoons per day) than dozens of pills, and it's far more effective. It is even able to kill parasites that don't respond to any other treatments.

One of my clients, Mrs. Sellers, has been covered with body sores and rashes for years. They were diagnosed as hookworms that her body encased in the scabs on her skin, but no medicine was able to kill them. She is now delighted to see them clearing with the Copper Solution.

I saw the same thing on a patient in the emergency room at the hospital where I did my clinical studies for Emergency Medical Training class. I tried to tell the doctor what it was, but he laughed me off. Thought I was a nut for even suggesting to use ... *copper*? Sad to say, his patient certainly didn't get the help he needed. What was even sadder, the patient's wife is now also breaking out with them.

Earl and his wife in Texas had a recurring problem with parasites that nothing could eliminate. They had spent a small fortune running from one medical parasite specialist to another, but to no avail. I sent him the Copper Solution, and with only thirty-two ounces, it is gone. He had also been in the Middle East for some time, where we see a very strange parasite in those coming from the Middle East or Far Eastern countries. It is white and about one foot long with a black head. The copper even kills that one.

The parasites are often hard to see because the feces will wrap around the dead ones and carry them out of the body. One of my clients in Hillsboro, Oregon, is a nurse. She swore that she didn't have parasites but (as unpleasant as this seems) when she broke apart her stools, she very quickly filled a quart jar with parasites she never knew she had.

It has been my experience that nearly everyone reaches a point in their recovery when they pass an orange worm. It is usually nine to twelve inches long, flat and paper thin (about one-quarter inch wide). When I first saw it, I thought I had swallowed a sliver of carrot that just hadn't digested, until it dawned on me that I would never swallow a slice of carrot that large. In talking to some of my other clients, they related similar experiences. Not long ago, I was reading a book on Indian folk medicine. What a surprise to read about them in there. They related that they knew a person was going to get well when they passed the "Orange Worm." The description fit exactly what we had experienced. It was just another confirmation that I was on the right track and well on the road to complete recovery.

At the beginning of Step Two, I also recommend starting with a product called Noni, a plant grown in the organic lava beds of Hawaii. It is a wonderful plant that does so many special things. It stops the growth of the K-Ras (early) cancer cells, kills some parasites, and boosts the immune system. It's a proxeronine, a substance that stimulates the body's production of xeronine, an alkaloid needed to repair the RNA of cells and cell walls. (This will be explained more fully in the next chapter when I talk about fibromyalgia.) This herb has done wonders to speed up the program for our clients, sometimes cutting their recovery time in half.

For the first ten days, the program is limited to the Liver/Gall Bladder Formula, Copper Solution, and Noni. If we don't proceed slowly, your body will react too fast and you'll get so sick that you won't be able to work or do much of anything. Most of my clients have to keep working but, by going slowly, they are able to handle the program.

STEP THREE

By day 15, most of the parasites should be gone, and the liver should be working at a much greater efficiency. So now that the body is able to begin getting the full benefit of the proper nutrients, we can start rebuilding the immune system. This is vital to prevent the diseases from coming back and to continue toward full recovery.

When I speak about the immune system, I am primarily referring to the thymus gland and the body's ability to make T cells. What I am going to explain now is an oversimplification of the immune system. It is in no way intended to be a complete study, but I hope to convey enough to you that you will understand what is basically going on in your body and what needs to be corrected. When most people talk about the immune system, they are talking about the lymph glands. I don't believe this is the immune system, but is really more the sewer system of the body. It carries waste from the cells to the spleen to be eliminated through proper processes. It also houses some of the immune cells, but they are not made there.

All immune cells are manufactured in the bone. Half of them mature in the bone and are called B cells. These go from the marrow of the bone directly into the bloodstream and lymph glands where they become our first line of defense—our ground troops, so to speak. They go after bacteria and any normal invader of the body, killing it off. These are the defenders that can kill some of the cells containing the normal viruses, too, but are not able to kill cellular diseases.

BONE

T Cells	B Cells

Lymph Glands (Sewer System of Body)
Exercise is the pump for lymph glands

Blood Stream
Heart is the pump for bloodstream

B Cells *First line of defense;*
Kill bacteria and most common viruses

T Cells *Eat tumors, tuberculosis, cancer,*
skin eruptions

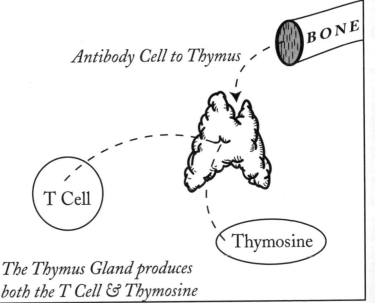

Antibody Cell to Thymus

BONE

T Cell

Thymosine

The Thymus Gland produces
both the T Cell & Thymosine

The other half of our antibodies are manufactured in the bone, but travel to the thymus gland, which is located about an inch below the point of the collarbone. There they are converted into T cells, designed to eat cellular diseases such as cancer, tumors, tuberculosis, and skin eruptions, but are still not able to do their job. They are spread throughout the body, waiting to be "told" what to do. You can find pictures of them in just about any high-school or college biology book, which shows the matured or coded ones eating diseased tissue.

The thymus gland also puts out a hormone called thymosine. This is the computer system of the body, for it travels throughout the systems, looking for diseased tissue. When it finds it, it then locates a T cell, codes it to kill that particular kind of cell by putting a "receptor" on it and goes on about its business. It is like an army general tagging the soldiers he wants to go into battle, then sending them out with specific orders. Once that T cell is coded (for example, it may be coded to kill a kaposi sarcoma), it can then only kill that kind of cancer and no other. It will find one and eat it.

Because of its ability to do only a specific job, a fresh supply of new T cells is always in demand. That is why it is so necessary to restore the thymus gland, so there will be plenty to do whatever job is needed.

If a doctor tells you that you have cancer but have a healthy immune system, that is just not so. If you did, then your body could produce enough T cells to eat all the cancer cells in the body, keeping the disease in check. Science looks at the tumor and tries to kill it, using its poisons to kill the good T cells at the same time without trying to help the body restore the thymus gland and T-cell production. No wonder they can only tell you it is in remission. They have done nothing to prevent it from growing again.

A couple of years ago, I spoke with some researchers in France who were working on the AIDS problem. We talked about thymosine, and when I asked if they knew anything about its function, they said yes. They have increased it in the peripheral bloodstream of AIDS patients, and observed that the disease immediately backed down or decreased.

So I asked them if they were then trying to restore the thymus gland so the body could produce its own thymosine. They laughed at me and said, "Why would we want to do that? That gland only regulates the rate of growth of the child. It isn't even needed in the adult."

I was flabbergasted that this AIDS researcher—who had just told me that thymosine is made in the thymus gland and is important in killing AIDS—would say that restoring this gland was of no interest to his colleagues! I sat there, looking at my college biology book that said the thymus gland made T cells to eat cellular diseases—and this scientist said it wasn't important? I was totally baffled.

To determine if a person has AIDS, medical science does a CD4, T-cell count to determine the level of T cells in the blood. It should be between 880 and 1,200. If it is about 500 or lower, the person is told they have AIDS, whether or not they are HIV positive.

Yet everyone who has *any major disease* will also have a T-cell count that is *way below normal or even nonexistent.* Why don't they tell *them* that they have AIDS?

I believe we are again being handed a lot of medical double talk. I have had so many of my clients ask their doctors for a CD4 test, but almost every time, they are refused. Why? I think it is because doctors have developed tunnel vision concerning their approach to disease treatment. Chemicals have become the cure-all. I don't think they are even taught prevention or how to measure a person's immunity levels.

Case in point: In August 1998, Bruce from Vancouver, Washington, came to talk to me about his cancer. He is in his early 40s, a father to young children and has a lot to live for. He had been diagnosed with colon cancer and had already gone through chemo and surgery to remove the tumor and insert a colostomy. Several months later, he went for a checkup, only to learn that the tumor was back and now the size of his fist.

A mutual friend, Leslie, told him how she and several of her friends had used my products to remove tumors and get well. Because chemo and surgery didn't stop the disease the first time, he decided to try the herbal route instead. He started the program and, much to the joy of his family, when he went back to check on the colostomy in midwinter, the tumor was gone and the colostomy could be removed.

As of March 1999, he has returned to work and is living a full, active life. I encouraged him to stay on the program until his CD4 test showed him that his immune system is strong enough to prevent the cancer from coming back.

He had his doctor call me to give me the test results. When he read me the report, he said that Bruce's T-cell count was normal (at 400?). He didn't even realize that that is a dangerously low count. Now, if they had been suspicious that he had HIV, they would have immediately declared that he had AIDS. But because he had cancer, they said the count was ... *normal?* I have a hard time understanding their thinking. But I'm very glad that Bruce is staying with the program until his T-cell count is as high as it can go (to 1,200).

When I realized I needed to keep track of my CD4 count, I had already been on the program, especially the Immune

Formula, for a couple of years. My count was 890, but now, two years later, it is 1,050. I wish I had known about this test when I was really ill. It would have been nice to have had the numbers for comparison.

CD4 T-Cell Count: 800–1,200

So, on day 15, we add the immune formula to rebuild your T-cell count so you can stay well. Stay with it until your count is at or near 1,200. Then you are safe. At this point, the program is limited to the Liver/Gallbladder Formula, Noni, Copper Solution and Immune Formula.

STEP FOUR

Now for the last step. Starting on day 26, we add the Herbal Extract to kill off the remaining cancer cells and viruses. We start with only one drop a day for the first week, two drops a day for the second week, and so on until you are taking at least ten drops a day until you are well and your T cell count is back to normal. Some people are so sick, they can't even increase a drop a week, but increase only as they are able. When added to an eight-ounce glass of cranberry or aronia berry juice that is slowly sipped throughout the day, or taken with meals, most people can tolerate the extract with no problem.

Cleansing and rebuilding your system to get rid of disease and prevent further illness is a slow process. It takes at least three months to regrow tissue or organs, so stay with it. The rewards are worth it. When your immune system is strong, no matter what comes your way, it is your best defense. You will then be living a full, healthy life and LIVING FREE of disease.

Chapter 9

TAKING CARE OF
YOUR LOVED ONES

S ome of my greatest rewards have come from watching the
joy that people experience as they see their loved ones get
well. This is especially true when I am able to help children live
full, healthy lives, so they can realize their dreams. There have
been some very hard times over the past ten years, but knowing
I have made a difference in people's lives makes it all worth-
while.

The failures have been hard to take but, unfortunately, failure is a part of life and a part of learning. I have tried many,
many products in my search for answers—products everyone
touted as the *answer,* the *cure-all.* But most of these products
were dismal failures. If they didn't work at least 75 percent of
the time, I discarded them from the program.

There are a lot of wonderful products and many well-
meaning people selling them, but they have only parts of the
picture. If you grow up eating nothing but junk food, and suddenly you decide to eat fresh vegetables, of course you will feel
better. For the first time in your life, you are actually feeding
your body.

This is what happens to a lot of people who suddenly start
taking a good cell food, a good vitamin, a good mineral and
such. They feel great, so they go off the deep end and think that
that one product is the cure-all because it did so much for them.

For others who have practiced good nutrition and taken supplements all their lives, when they get sick, it takes more.

With the Four-Step Program, I have endeavored to reach all of you, whether you have practiced good nutrition or not. Therefore, I tested many of the so-called cures for years. The only ones I have kept in the program are the ones that worked for everyone, no matter what their nutritional habits have been.

In the health-food industry, as in other industries, fads run wild. Among the most recent are chondroitin sulfate and glucosamine. Suddenly it is THE treatment for all arthritic and joint pain, and now everyone is selling it. All you have to do is attend one of the alternative-healing fairs, and you will see 95 percent of the booths claiming that their products are unique, the best.

But if you look at the product labels, you'll see that they are all selling variations of the same thing. Most of them are touting weight-loss programs, ways to get your youth back by taking their product, which they guarantee will turn back your biological clock. Some are just outright charlatans and in it for the money. The search for the Fountain of Youth is just as much alive today as it was in the days of Ponce de León.

I had a booth at one such fair in Los Angeles recently, and out of the more than a hundred booths, there were no more than fifteen that really sold something helpful. I accidentally walked into a lecture being given by a man selling rods that emit a heat and light frequency. I nearly choked when he told people they could insert this rod rectally, and the heat from it would cure their colon cancer.

Later, I took a good look at his material and claims. Believe me, if I had used that hot rod up my "you know what," after you peeled me off the ceiling I doubt I'd be any better at all. The real heartbreak was talking with a woman and her daughter who both had cancer. They stopped at my booth and told me that they'd already done chemo and radiation, but to no avail. Now they had bought this man's story, and his products, and left.

Unfortunately, that kind of product gives us all bad reputations.

That experience reminded me that there are some good, caring doctors out there who have a real heart for people. I know because I had two uncles that were, and I know quite a few of them who are not afraid to step out of the norm and stand up for what they believe is right—even in the face of reprisal from the medical board.

Unfortunately, the money to be gained by the doctors, hospitals and pharmaceutical companies overshadow them—just as the large number of those involved with fads and cure-alls in the alternative field overshadow those of us who love God, care about people, and are trying to do an honest job.

God is my judge and my source of life and income. I don't need to sell you products to get wealthy. My Father owns the cattle on a thousand hills and all the gold in the richest mines in the world. Because you are His child, as I am, you deserve the best He has for us, and that is honesty. I give you my pledge, that to the best of my ability, with God's help, you will always get that from me.

Illness changes even the most wonderful people. There are some common reactions or problems in almost everyone who is experiencing a major illness that usually even they are not aware of. It is my hope that by understanding what to expect from your loved one or friend, it will help you cope with their reactions.

If you can learn to step out of the situation and understand that they are not attacking *you*, it will help you deal with their outbursts. First, the person becomes irritable and irrational. The normally sweet human being you have known and loved for so long gradually changes. They snap at you, and later vehemently deny it. They slam out of the house, cry at the drop of a hat, display incredible mood swings from hopefulness to despair (often within minutes), and become a demanding, self-centered monster that you feel you don't even know anymore.

If you take their actions personally, you too will ride an emotional roller coaster that you'll desperately want to get off. Realize that these behaviors are NORMAL for this person, at this time. So try to focus on the person you knew and loved, not on the one they've become. Be as loving, supportive and as non-combative as you possibly can and PRAY A LOT.

When it gets to be too much, quietly arrange to get away for awhile and take a personal break. Go to a funny movie, read a funny book, or as I do, go to the store and spend a long time reading funny greeting cards or browsing through magazines. Or go for a long walk or a swim at the pool. It is an effort to make yourself do it, but if you do something to treat yourself and relax, you will be able to cope much better.

Second—and probably hardest—is helping to keep the sick person from giving up. I cannot tell you how many people with major illnesses just can't hang on to hope and give up. When illness strikes, it doesn't just strike the body, but it also hits hard on the emotions, making it nearly impossible for them to keep a positive attitude.

So help them concentrate on God, the true source of their healing, and on His provision for their journey back. When a person is told they have a major disease like cancer or Lou Gehrig's disease, they go through the normal steps of, first, denial, then bargaining, then fear, and finally acceptance.

TAKING CARE OF YOUR LOVED ONES

I once knew a young mother of two small children in Cincinnati, Ohio, who was told she only had only a few months to live because she had developed cancer. She looked the doctor in the eye and said, "That's what you think. I have small children to raise, and *I* am going to raise them. Not somebody else." With that, she stomped out of the office and, twenty-five years later, is still going strong.

Yet you see others who accept defeat just by the implication of "the disease," and they give up before they even try. Many will say they are fighting the disease, but their subconscious has heard the big "C" word and tells the person, even though they don't realize it, that this is a deadly disease and they will die. Their subconscious finally overcomes their conscious efforts, and they lose the battle.

Time and time again, I have seen a person either get well physically or be clearly on the road to recovery, and then they suddenly stop the program. You must find out why they got sick to start with (this will be covered in more depth in the next chapter), and help them overcome that issue, or you will not be able to stop the disease.

We experienced a prime example of this kind of thing with one of my clients from Washington. When I first talked to her, she was suffering from throat cancer. She had stopped smoking, but was on oxygen and experiencing a great deal of pain. I started her on the Herbal Extract, making sure she drank it slowly to allow the extract plenty of time to get to the tumors down her throat. Within days, she started experiencing a gagging feeling, after which she would cough up small tumors that had come loose from the wall of her throat.

Finally, all the tumors were out, she was off the oxygen, and was well on her way to a full recovery. Then, for no reason anyone could figure out, she stopped taking everything and went back to smoking. She refused help to find out why, and eventually died of lung cancer. This is not an isolated case, but all too often true when people refuse to deal with the spiritual and emotional causes for their illness.

Here lies your biggest battle: I knew a 12-year-old youth in Oregon who had leukemia. His mom believed in alternative treatments, but the courts took him away from her because she didn't want him to have chemo and radiation. She never refused him care, but she wanted to use alternatives for a more natural approach.

The only way she could get him back was to do what the courts said, which included that they would not allow her to use nutritional supplements of any kind or any alternative treatment. It had to be strictly what they approved and nothing else.

It was heart-rending to watch this mother suffer along with the boy. Unbeknowns to the doctors, she did give him natural supplements along with what they were mandating. But sadly, it was too late. The boy became so sick and so tired of taking so many pills, that he finally said, "No more." No amount of coaxing would change his mind. I couldn't figure out why the courts were so adamant that she do only what they wanted. Eventually, the boy died.

That was when they told her the truth. The medical community was experimenting with a new cancer-treatment drug and wanted to know if or how it would work, and any other treatment would alter their results. They said they knew he was going to die anyway, so they didn't think they were doing anything wrong. It was for the benefit of mankind.

What about the benefit of this boy and the mother who loved him so much—and about *his* chance for life? What about the emotional trauma that this terribly sick, frightened little boy suffered by being wrenched from his mother's arms—the ones he needed most for comfort—only to be placed in a sterile hospital room, where they made him even sicker with their "treatments"?

Only God can heal the inner man, but your love and support are vital to the person's total recovery. Here is where you become God's hand to them.

Control stress around anyone who is ill and in your own life. Stress is a very toxic emotion that wipes out our immune systems and our ability to fight.

«IDD»

Immune-Deficient Diseases

---

1. Thyroid

2. Goiter

3. Allergies

4. Asthma

5. Diabetes

6. Cancer

7. AIDS

8. Tumors

Chapter 10

MORE CASE HISTORIES

The following information is to give you an understanding of what I found helpful in working with victims of various illnesses. I have found that sick people have a great deal of trouble following even the simplest directions, so I have laid out the program on a blue chart form to keep track of what they do and when. It is a guide only, not an absolute that you must follow every day. With some people, the disease is so pervasive they have to go extremely slow or they will feel so sick that they either give up or can't function. The program is designed to avoid this, so only increase to the next step when you feel you can handle it.

AIDS

Acquired Immune Deficiency Syndrome (AIDS) is not caused by a virus, whether it is HIV or any other virus, and researchers have never proved that it is. Because so many people are infected by the HIV retrovirus (see Chapter 8), science assumes that it causes AIDS. Since millions of people got the polio shot containing the Simian 40 virus—which often shows up as HIV—why wouldn't it be present in so many people who get AIDS?

By assuming that a virus causes AIDS is just as logical as saying that because most redheads have fair skin and burn easily, we can assume that red hair causes the sun to burn them.

One of the reasons researchers may believe a virus causes AIDS is because the virus attacks the matured T cells, enters it through the receptor, bonds with the RNA of that cell and tricks it into thinking it is an HIV virus, changing the makeup of the cell wall. It then becomes a manufacturing plant for HIV. It also attacks the thymus gland, rendering it useless for thymosine production and for making more T cells.

HIV Contributes to AIDS But Doesn't Cause It

How HIV attacks the T cell as it spreads from host to host.

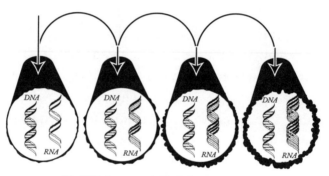

The HIV virus enters the T cell through the receptor.

There are hundreds of people who have AIDS yet are not HIV positive. Thousands and thousands more have HIV, but not AIDS. They have no explanation for it, but continue to lie to us saying that HIV causes AIDS.

Science tells those in the natural-food business that we aren't valid because we don't do blind studies and spend millions of dollars pursuing laboratory results to get FDA approval.

In fact, that same group that approves chemicals and drugs like Phen Phen, without making sure they are safe, has the audacity to assume HIV causes AIDS and touts that as truth? Where is their laboratory proof? Why are we wrong because we

140

don't have laboratory evidence yet why are they right to allow products like Phen Phen when they didn't have proof it was safe? AIDS is simply a loss of the immune system, which can happen by drug use, exposure to chemicals, living a promiscuous lifestyle, and so on. If you think that giving drug addicts clean needles is going to stop AIDS, well, I have a bridge in Brooklyn I'll sell you real cheap.

The use of drugs destroys the body, the immune system and life itself. But AIDS isn't a virus that clean needles will stop.

The government would like you to believe AIDS is caused by a sexually transmitted virus called HIV, when in reality, that is not true. If you will look in high-school and college biology books, you will learn that they have found HIV present IN ALL BODY FLUIDS, including tears and perspiration. In fact, it has been proven that it is found in higher concentration in the saliva and urine than it is in the blood.

Years ago Dr. Lorraine Day, an orthopedic surgeon at the Medical Teaching Hospital in San Francisco, tried to tell them HIV was present in blood. They attempted to destroy her for telling the truth and for trying to warn health-care practitioners to wear protection when coming into contact with their patient's blood. They swore that it was just present in seminal or vaginal fluids—only to have to admit to us later that indeed it was in blood. The story is related in Dr. Day's book, *AIDS: What the Government Isn't Telling You.*

Next they tried to tell us for years that you can only get it if you have a blood transfusion, have blood spilled on an open wound, or have sexual relations with an infected individual. All three are lies and I'll tell you why.

First, this is not a sexually transmitted disease (STD) like gonorrhea, chlamydia, genital herpes or syphilis. These bacteria or viruses only live in vaginal or seminal fluids while HIV lives in ANY body fluid. Telling you and your children to have "safe" sex by using a condom is playing Russian roulette because the pores of a condom are three microns wide. A virus is less than one micron wide, so how can a condom prevent you from getting a sexually transmitted virus? This is like going down to the ocean, lining the shore with giant sponges, and thinking it will hold back a tidal wave. What a ludicrous, dangerous lie.

A condom doesn't even stop pregnancy 35 percent of the time. If a condom has been exposed to heat or smog anywhere in the shipping process, it breaks down even more. The condom manufacturers profit big time from that masterful piece of propaganda, and we bought it hook, line and sinker. Ask any high-school student and their "health" teacher. Besides, since HIV is present in all body fluids, how about its transmission during heavy kissing, which often causes broken capillaries in the mouth?

Second, your skin has millions of receptors that catch and draw in things you apply to it. For instance, heart patients wear nitroglycerine patches so they can absorb it through their skin and get what their heart needs at any time. Women with hormone deficiencies wear estrogen patches. When you look at how tiny a virus is and the fact that the skin has receptors to grab it, what makes you think you can't get a virus this way?

At the same time that government agencies said you can't get the HIV virus through the skin, the courts proved the opposite. Last year, in Portland, Oregon, a man was convicted of attempted murder because he tried to give a police officer HIV by spitting on him. Did the court just think he wasn't a nice guy and wanted to get him for attempted murder? If the prosecution hadn't proved that it was possible to get HIV through saliva applied to the skin, then why was he convicted of attempted murder? Am I missing something here? Do I just not "get" the medical profession's story?

Or could it be that we have been duped?

If you believe as I do—that AIDS is a loss of the IMMUNE SYSTEM and is not a virus—then you will also believe it is curable. I have no doubt that the HIV virus does exist in many people, and that it contributes to AIDS because it destroys T cells and the thymus gland. But I do not believe that HIV causes AIDS.

When AIDS first surfaced, it was called the gay cancer. For years, they tried to say it was spread through the gay community because it's a virus. The gay lobbyists want to find a virus because, if they do, a vaccine could be developed and they wouldn't have to change their lifestyle. But it isn't a virus that causes AIDS. It's their practices that cause AIDS.

When you study the Four-Step Program, you realize the importance of the health of the liver. Ninety percent of the gay community is infected with hepatitis, which destroys that processing plant. In addition to the practice of "fisting," you realize that their immune systems are already in trouble. Also, rectal sex tears the delicate colon tissue, allowing feces to enter the bloodstream. Feces is such a toxic waste that when it is used for fertilizer, as the Koreans do, you can get amoebic dysentery that nothing cures.

Again, quotes from Dr. Gallo and Hanna Kroeger, respectively:

> My new co-worker Anita Agarwal, working with Veffa Franchini, discovered that two parasites found in fecal material, giardia and amoeba, can be infected in HIV. These parasites are not uncommon in Central Africa and in gay men

everywhere. We wonder whether this is a factor in HIV communicability.

In the presence of parasites, retrovirus takes on the form of HIV. According to the findings of Dr. Gallo and associates, the co-factor that changes retrovirus into action to become HIV is parasitic poisons: amoeba, hookworm, and giardia. I suggest that in any case the entire body should be treated by eliminating the lesser evils and counteracting the retrovirus at the same time.

I couldn't agree with them more.

Along with their practice of "ringing," "golden showers" and so on, they spread parasites and definitely destroy the immune system. STDs are so prevalent in that community that antibiotics are used on a regular basis. It is common knowledge that overuse of antibiotics is detrimental to your health. If someone isn't willing to change the lifestyle that gave them AIDS to start with, then I usually discourage them from purchasing our products because I feel it is a waste of their money. If change is their desire, then we can help them.

The following are stories of three of the many clients we have helped.

Peter and Tom, both from New York, had AIDS. They followed the blue program sheet for several months, eventually dropping everything except the Immune Formula. Their T-cell count came back up from below 500 to reach 1,200, a high normal, where it still remains three years later. Their doctor—who had been checking their T-cell count for several years and treating them with AZT (which literally eats T cells) and all kinds of experimental drugs—checked their nearly normal counts, and responded like so many do by saying, "Gee, we must have misdiagnosed you to start with."

MORE CASE HISTORIES

Another case, Kelly from California, was diagnosed with AIDS and a T-cell count of below 30. He was skin and bones, couldn't eat much, and was so weak that taking a shower and shaving exhausted him so completely that he had to sleep for three hours to get enough energy to do anything else. He started on our Four-Step's blue program forms around Christmas 1996.

Within twenty-four hours of starting the parasite program, he was famished. He ate everything he could get his hands on. He even got up in the middle of the night to go out and get a hamburger. He rapidly gained weight and strength. By March, he was traveling all over the country, enjoying a full life and planning a week-long backpacking trip on horses in Portugal.

Everyone around him knew what he was doing, even his doctor. He called me one day to tell me that he was anemic and the doctors wanted to do a blood transfusion. I begged him not to do that, explaining that the high volume of parasites he had had caused this. I urged him instead to go with the natural approach of taking our Iron Water, hematinics (capsules high in iron and B vitamins), a homeopathic called ferrum phos, which helps absorb iron, and to eat foods high in iron such as eggs, liver and sweet potatoes.

About a week later, a mutual friend called to ask if there was anything I could do to help him because the doctors had talked him into having a blood transfusion, which they later learned was infected with lupus. How could they *not know* the blood was tainted when it had been tested? I was told that the doctors put him on drugs to suppress the liver and the immune system, and had assigned nurses to take care of him around the clock to be sure he took the drugs they prescribed. In three weeks, he was dead. What a waste. He was such a wonderful young man.

One final thing before I leave the subject of AIDS. I believe that many men think they are homosexual because they feel feminine and drawn to men. But in reality, they are just over-loaded with female hormones. In my experience, I have found the large majority of gay men are heavy meat eaters, and meat is LOADED WITH FEMALE HORMONES. Most meat companies use them while the animals are being fattened for market because the hormones make their muscles flabby, which causes the meat to be more tender, and help build fat and weight.

I was in Puerto Rico for a dog show a few years ago and noticed more gay men per capita than I ever saw anywhere else I had traveled (and I've traveled the world a lot). I thought something was wrong, but didn't know what, until a week or two after I got home. I was watching a "20/20" pro-gram in which they talked about the problems surfacing in Puerto Rico. They noticed that 4- and 5-year-old girls were developing breasts and having menstrual cycles. When they took them off meats, they went back to normal. The govern-ment checked the meats and found the female-hormone level to be extremely high. This, along with what I observed myself, makes me believe that the high amount of female hormones in meat is making "gays" out of guys who aren't. I wonder how many of them would love to know their emo-tional and behavioral problems are caused from the meats they eat?

Recently, I completed training for EMT Basic (Emergency Medical Technician), and was surprised to learn how they approach exposure to HIV. They put EMTs on leave, start them on AZT (which literally eats the very T cells they are trying to protect), and do periodic blood tests.

This is archaic and so misleading. Once you have been exposed to the HIV virus, it could take up to ten years before the body produces antibodies to it. This is called the "open-window effect." You could be full of the virus, but your body is not able to react and build antibodies, especially if your immune system is low. So you could test negative when, in reality, you are carrying it.

If you are ever exposed to the HIV virus and want to be tested, make sure they use the P24 test, which actually tests for the presence of the virus itself. That will tell you immediately if you have been exposed.

The Four-Step Program should address all the problems you may encounter with this disease. YOU CAN FULLY RECOVER.

ALLERGIES AND HYPOTHYROID

Allergies and hypothyroid conditions are both immune-deficient diseases. In every case where we have put the person on the Immune Formula, the thyroid has been corrected in about three months. Allergies take longer, but in time, most people experience relief. Yet in order to clear them, you MUST build the immune system.

Most doctors will have you running for allergy shots, but I believe you should instead restore the root problem, the immune system. I used to be so allergic to cigarettes that I would sometimes end up on oxygen during a long flight. Although I usually flew at night to avoid the heavy smokers, and always sat in the no-smoking section, the smoke was in the filter system, so I still suffered. But now that the Immune Formula has restored my immune system, I can be around cigarettes for a while before they bother me (even though I still find them unpleasant).

I also took Thyroxin for thirty-five years for a hypothyroid. But once the formula also corrected my thyroid, I went hyperthyroid until I stopped the Thyroxin.

Asthma

Asthma is also an allergy-related disease. My sister Martha suffered from it all her life. I can remember as a child, rushing her to the hospital to get adrenaline shots so she wouldn't choke to death. I can't remember a time when she was able to sleep lying flat because, if she did, she couldn't get her breath. She was never without her atomizer. I developed the Lung and Joint Formula for her. It was a joy to see her be able to take and be more comfortable, even able to go out occasionally without the atomizer. It is called Lung and Joint because these are basically connected. If someone has a lung problem, he or she usually experiences joint swelling and pain.

For treatment, follow the blue form, but go very slowly to give the body time to dump the waste buildup in your system. This may mean that you start with only half a capsule of Liver Formula until you can tolerate it, then go to one and gradually increase until you're up to dose. Do the same thing with the Immune Formula because the lymph glands dump partially through the lungs. If you start to get congestion from the liver or immune system dumping too fast, don't increase your dosage until you are comfortable at the level where you first began to experience problems. Instead of increasing according to the program, only progress to the next step as you feel better.

Alzheimer's Disease and Dementia

One of my clients, a physician from Texas, believes as I do that there is a virus connected to both of these. His mother, who was 85-years-young at the time, was in a nursing home and combative, incoherent and incontinent. They wanted to put her on antidepressants and keep her sedated, but this doctor would not hear of it. He put her on our Kidney/Bladder, Nerve and Muscle, Herbal Extract (to kill the virus) and Liver formulas.

148

In three weeks, she was at home, totally coherent and continent. She was her old self. He called me to tell me what had happened and said the only thing wrong was that she just wouldn't stop talking!

I believe there are a lot of parasites involved with Alzheimer's, too, but I haven't been able to find anyone who is willing to test the program. I believe this because of an experience related to me by a doctor here in Portland, Oregon. She said she had been in Central America for several years with her husband, who was in the military. She visited a local hospital where she saw a man acting exactly the same way an advanced-Alzheimer's patient acts.

When she inquired as to the reason why, they informed her that he had a parasite in his brain, but they couldn't remove it or kill it. He was going to die, they said, but they didn't believe he was in any pain. He definitely didn't know anyone around him, where he was, or what was happening to him.

Is there a connection? Do we ever treat an Alzheimer's patient for parasites? No, we're ignoring this problem in just about everybody, much less victims of Alzheimer's. Why can't science look for the more obvious instead of always looking for some exotic cause?

ARTHRITIS AND CHRONIC PAIN

This is absolutely curable and has been for over twenty-seven years, but the medical profession has had the cure and kept it under wraps. Since they are so heavily tied in with the pharmaceutical companies, is it any wonder? They make billions of dollars from medicines that control arthritis pain. Do you honestly believe they want you to get cured? If you do, I still have that bridge for sale.

The patent on one product has now been removed, making it available to the general public. It is called cetyl-myristoleate and it works. Joyce, in Indiana, suffered from rheumatoid arthritis for many years. Her hands were so crippled she could barely hold a hairbrush or a pen. She needed help dressing and doing most simple tasks. She was so bad she needed three bottles (most people only need one or two bottles) of the Artho-Flex containing cetyl-myristoleate to clear it.

Recently, Joyce left a message on my answering machine ordering other products. Her closing comment was "If you need to talk to me, you can call me—but don't call between 7 and 9 p.m. because I'll be at my line-dancing class." I spoke to her daughter recently who told me she was totally cleared of the arthritis. They are thrilled. Her recovery is very typical of the response we get.

The nice thing is that once these clients are cleared, they don't need the product anymore. Is it any wonder the medical community doesn't want this product widely used? They can't mass produce it chemically to gain great profits because it is a natural substance extracted from beef tallow and natural cow's butter—two things they are telling us to eliminate from our diets.

There were some that had experienced relief, but not completely. I was sitting one day, praying and asking God what to do for those suffering from chronic pain and for others who didn't get completely well. I felt that He was telling me to combine the Nerve and Muscle Formula with equal amounts of cetyl-myristoleate. It didn't make sense to me because I'd used them at the same time but hadn't seen much response.

But again, I felt the urge to do it. Since I've learned to listen to that voice, I decided to try blending them. The response has been phenomenal. When the new product, Nerve and

Muscle Plus, was taken along with the Artho-Flex, almost immediately the stubborn pain subsided.

Voilà! Score another one for God.

Ruth, who works for me, has had arthritis in her toes for years. The only way she could get around was when her feet became numb. She'd taken the Artho-Flex, which started to clear the arthritis, but then her feet lost their numbness and began to hurt so badly she had to stop. She decided to try two capsules of Nerve and Muscle Plus when she went to bed. She said she figured she had nothing to lose, so why not?

When she awoke in the morning, she immediately noticed she was able to totally feel her feet, but there was NO PAIN. Later in the day, she realized she was no longer feeling the pain in her hip and ribcage. Even the pain she'd been treating in her injured upper-left arm WAS GONE.

I had twisted my right foot and snapped a small bone on top (which now protrudes). The pain was intense, especially after I'd drive for awhile. One evening I decided to try the new formula and, much to my delight, within two hours the pain was gone and has never come back! My desk sits in a draft that no one has been able to stop. The draft goes right across my legs and, after a few months of winter, created a chronic aching of my leg muscles. Within three days of starting this formula, the stiffness and aching disappeared.

One day I was chatting with Brenda, a friend of mine, who told me that she and her husband were suffering from incredible back pain. They had to start moving in a few days, but she was dreading it. She just didn't know how they were going to be able to load the heavy animal cages, furniture and such with as much pain as they were having. I sent her a bottle of the Nerve and Muscle Plus. She was delighted. They took two the evening it arrived, and two the next morning. Nearly all the pain was gone within a few hours, in spite of loading all day. It has continued to give them both relief.

At the publishing of this book, we are testing Nerve and Muscle Plus with migraine headaches and are having great success. Three or four capsules used at the onset of a migraine headache seem to stop the migraine. (Magnesium Water also greatly relieves migraines.)

The only people who have not experienced pain relief with the formula are those with ruptured discs in their back, while foot pain or numbness seem always to go away.

BLOOD PRESSURE IRREGULARITIES, CHOLESTEROL CARDIAC PROBLEMS

Many in my family have either died of heart attacks or have had open-heart surgery. I decided to develop a formula that would keep this from happening to me, thus the Heart and Blood Vessel Formula came into existence. After I took the diet pill Phen Phen, I developed an irregular heart rate (an extra beat just before it was supposed to). After a trip to the emergency room, where I was told that this type of irregularity is not life threatening, I started taking my own formula. Within minutes, my heart calmed down and went back to normal. The irregular heartbeat still returns periodically, but all I have to do is take one pill, twice daily for a day or two, and it corrects.

Sandy, a client in California, has too many nerves going to her heart (her father also has the same genetic problem). If she exercised at all by taking a walk near Lake Tahoe in the mountains—or even thought about it—or watched a thriller movie, her heart started beating at double the normal rate, and she'd end up in intensive care at the hospital.

She heard about the Heart and Blood Vessel Formula and decided to try it, instead of cutting the extra nerve. On just two capsules a day of all-natural, herbal and glandular ingredients, both she and her dad are living full, normal lives with a normal heart rate.

I have had MANY clients come with high cholesterol and either high or low blood pressure. Many are taking medications that have bad side effects such as impotency, inability to sleep at night, restlessness, shortness of breath, and cataracts. After about 90 days on the Heart and Blood Vessel Formula, their blood pressure and cholesterol are normal or near normal with no side effects.

One thing to remember with any kind of serious heart problem is to start with chelation therapy to clean the blood vessels. Next, cut out oleo and margarine, which is nothing but the old lard game we did when I was a child. When we were poor, we couldn't afford butter, so my mom flavored the lard for us to use on our bread.

The only reason most of us in the natural-foods industry believe the American Heart Association tells you to eat margarine is because of margarine manufacturers, who stand to gain immense profits at your expense. Oleo, a hydrogenated oil that is turned into a saturated fat, is the worse thing you could eat if you have heart problems. You are better off eating real butter mixed with flaxseed oil, to keep the fat from settling in your blood vessels. It is easier for the body to process and besides, it contains the ingredient used in cetyl-myristoleate to cure arthritis.

The Heart and Blood Vessel Formula has even corrected cardiomyopathy.

CANCER

I have covered this topic quite a bit throughout the book, but will mention a few cases here. In dealing with nearly ten cases

T-Cell Coding

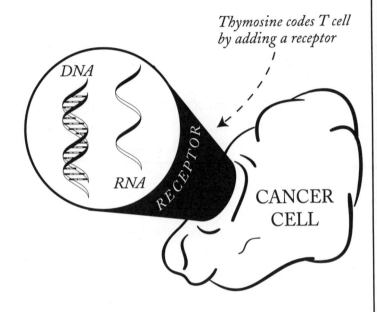

Thymosine codes T cell by adding a receptor

DNA

RNA

RECEPTOR

CANCER CELL

Two Types of Cancer

1. **Chemically Induced:** *Leukemia and inflammatory cancer caused by radiation, pesticide, herbicide, and chemical exposures.*

2. **Parasites:** *Tumors caused by threadworm, pinworm, cryptosporidium, and other foreign bodies.*

of cancer a day, I have found that cancer is a loss of the immune system, which allows the cells to grow unchecked. There are two forms of cancer: tumors (explained fully in Chapter 8), and interstitial, caused from exposure to chemicals such as pesticides, herbicides and radiation (leukemia is a good example).

Most people think that their cancer is different, and wonder if I've ever been able to help anyone with their particular kind of cancer (named according to where it attacks the body). My answer is, it doesn't make any difference where the cancer is, science doesn't treat it any differently (they use chemo and radiation for all of them). So why should I? The only adjustment we make is oxygenating the body more with lung and liver cancers. But for all cancers, we cleanse the body, rebuild it, kill off the cancer cells, and the body corrects itself.

I am appalled at the amount of surgery being done on men with prostate cancer. I have read and heard many reports that tell how just as many men survive without surgery as they do with surgery. There is no reason for any man to die of prostate cancer, for everyone that we have had on our program has recovered completely—without surgery.

Jim, in Idaho, had surgery, chemo, the whole barbaric route. But the count of his antibodies to prostate cancer (prostatic sensitivity antigen, or PSA) kept climbing. He came to me, and with only one bottle of Herbal Extract—and nothing else—his count was normal in just a few months.

Ira from Portland, Oregon, came to me with a high PSA, and didn't want to go the surgery route. I sold him some Herbal Extract and sent him to Dr. Abshier for follow-up. A few months later, he was well, healthy and his PSA was back to normal. I was stunned to hear that he then went back to his regular medical doctor for a checkup. This doctor talked him into surgery, even though he had been declared well! Unfortunately, this is all too common a scenario.

Brain tumors are fairly easy to eliminate because of the high blood flow. Stacey, in California, has a son named Shaun who developed a brain tumor when he was 7 years old. He had been on chemo, radiation, the whole nine yards, but the tumor kept growing. He was sleeping twenty hours each day, and was paralyzed on his left side.

In the fall of 1993, my friends started him on the Herbal Extract and the tumor began to shrink. When I met him in May 1994, he was well on his way to recovery. But we started him on the Immune and other products to make sure we got it all and that it would never come back. It has been some time since I talked to them, but they have continued to use the products. In March 1999, I met Shaun's dad, who was elated to see me. He said that Shaun had just celebrated his sixteenth birthday, there is no longer any sign of the tumor, and his son is the longest known survivor of this type of brain tumor. It looks like Shawn may well see his dreams for life come true.

I had a 24-year-old man from Vancouver, Washington, contact me because he had done everything he knew for his brain cancer. He had even gone to Mexico, but nothing was working. His mom purchased the program, but I didn't hear from them until April 1999, when she called to order some other products. When I asked how he was doing, she said, "Oh, he's fine. Completely cleared of any trace of cancer and back to work."

Glenn, in Portland, Oregon, had been using our products along with his wife who was suffering from multiple sclerosis. When she decided to do the parasite program, he felt that he should do it too, since he had never dewormed himself and wanted to be sure they were not passing them back and forth. He was also concerned because he was a smoker and several of his family members had died of lung cancer. As far as he knew, he didn't have it, but felt he should try anyway.

Fourteen days into the program, he started coughing up blood, so I advised him to go to a doctor. When they scoped him, they found that he had a small tumor in one lobe of the lung with a hole in it (where the parasite had come out and was now bleeding slightly). The doctors advised the usual chemo treatment, but he said no. He purchased a bottle of the Herbal Extract and a couple of weeks later, started gagging. He coughed up some dead tissue, and after that, he was fine. When his lungs were scoped again, the tumor was gone, and in its place was healthy pink tissue. Needless to say, he quit smoking and is now enjoying his retirement.

Sid, in his late 50s, of Vancouver, Washington, had an inoperable, untreatable non-Hodgkin's lymphoma, a cancer of the lymph cells, the variety caused from a T-cell disorder. According to the medical books, it is caused by an unknown retrovirus. Dr. Gallo says it is the Simian 40 virus. I believe Dr. Gallo, and believe it attacks the RNA of the lymph gland cells.

Since it is the same retrovirus, it should be approached the same way, so he started on the blue program sheet in November 1998. In April of 1999, we heard from him and his relatives that he is well.

Abe, from Ohio, is in his 80s and called me when he was diagnosed with inoperable bladder cancer. He was given six months to live, so he decided to try our program in June 1995. At this writing, he is still well and living a full, healthy life with no sign of cancer—and hasn't needed to use our products since 1997.

I have helped two gentlemen with sarcomas on their nose and face—Frank in California and Geary in Florida. In each case, the doctors wanted to remove half the face and do complete reconstructive surgery. They both opted to use my program by taking it internally to kill it from inside, and with a drop daily directly on the sarcoma. Each sarcoma was about the size of a fifty cent piece with fairly deep roots. Usually, the whole tumor will peel off within five days, and the skin will scab. But these tumors had deeper roots, so it took over a week for the tumors to come off. In both cases, after the tumor was off, there was a hole in the skin that did not bleed, eventually closed up, and left only a small scar.

We have literally hundreds of cases on file of cleared malignant and benign tumors.

CANDIDA

The intestinal tract must maintain a balance of good bacteria and yeast to have a healthy environment for foods to be properly digested. When you take antibiotics or go through a great deal of stress, the good bacteria are killed off, allowing the yeast to grow unchecked. The yeast then pushes through the intestinal wall into the bloodstream, where it breaks out in rashes and sores when it is deposited in the tissue, especially moist areas. Taking acidophilus helps restore the good bacteria to the intestinal tract, but you have to get it out of the rest of the body. The Herbal Extract drives it out of the tissue.

CEREBRAL PALSY

I have found two things that run common in those afflicted with this disease: They all have weakened immune systems and are allergic to sugar.

Carolyn in Oregon has a granddaughter about 5 years old with cerebral palsy (CP). She would stumble and fall, rolling as she did because she was unable to catch herself. She also had a terrible time sleeping, and woke up often, crying. She started on the Nerve and Muscle and Immune formulas, and within days she was sleeping through the night. In no time at all, she gained her balance, fell less and less, and caught herself when she did. Her improvement was remarkable, and then her mom took her off the products—why, no one can understand.

Another child, a 10-year-old who attends school with Leslie's daughter, had CP so badly she is wheelchair bound. She had to wear a bib because she drooled, couldn't talk, and definitely couldn't hold her own head up. Within just days of taking the Nerve and Muscle and Immune formulas, she was able to hold her head up by herself, stopped drooling, and began talking—and her mother took her off the products.

I can't imagine why some people do this, but this is fairly common with parents who have children suffering with this disease. Perhaps there is something psychological going on that they need to have their children dependent on them. I haven't figured it out yet.

Sara came to live with me when she was 10 years old. Diagnosed with CP, she had never been able to run and play; had to ascend or descend stairs one at a time, dragging her left leg; her left arm was nearly useless; and she was in a special-education class and labeled as learning disabled. She was born prematurely, and was a twin (her sibling didn't survive).

Sara had never eaten whole, fresh foods, and she lived on a high-sweets diet. I put her on the Immune, Nerve and Muscle, and Liver formulas, and in six months, you would never know she ever had CP. She now rollerblades, swims and runs with no problems. Within two days of removing sugar from her diet and adding fresh, whole foods and vegetables, her cognitive ability increased to a normal level. Today, three years later, she is now pulling straight A's and B's in normal classes in high school.

When I tried to help older people with CP, I found that we needed to start the program very slowly or they got so sick they'd quit. I think that is because they have had so many medications throughout the years that it is a fight to get their bodies cleaned up. And because their muscles have been weak for so long, it takes longer to get them back on their feet.

It is so hard for me to watch anyone suffering with this disease because I know it isn't necessary. I tried to give it to a local children's hospital—I was even willing to *donate* it—but they refused to even talk to me or let people know it is available. They thought it was wrong to promote a private company. It seems they would rather watch children suffer needlessly so they can promote drug companies—which offer CP patients no hope at all.

CHRONIC DEPRESSION AND CONSTIPATION

These are both linked to a congested liver. We have found that this clears up on the Liver/Gallbladder Formula. With depression, we also add the herbal Calmers. They really help one deal with fear, depression and anxiety.

Did you know that antidepressants can cause some people to become aggressive? Two of the boys who have been involved in shooting their classmates in the schools in the last year were taking antidepressants (Kip for seven years, and I don't know how long the other boy had been taking it).

Maybe we need to stop looking for other reasons for school violence and take another look at how we are treating teenage depression instead of handing this stuff out like it's as safe as candy!

CHRONIC FATIGUE, FIBROMYALGIA, AND EPSTEIN-BARR

All of these are caused from the Simian 40 retrovirus, which attacks muscle tissues. This is easily cleared with our program, and I have several cases to prove it. With this disease, it usually hits the hardest in your late 40s and up. Since it plugs up the cell walls, the more you exercise the weaker you get because you are using up nutrients your cells contain and can't get rid of the cell-waste buildup.

This is fairly easy to diagnose because of its distinct pain points on the outside of the elbows, knees, and heels, and on the back of the neck. Another clue to this condition can be, the more you exercise, the weaker you get. (I described many more symptoms when I talked about my own illness at the beginning of this book.)

Since the virus has invaded so much of the muscle tissue, you have to go slowly in killing it or you will not be able to function. Follow the blue program sheet, but go much slower with the Herbal Extract, usually staying on one or two drops for several weeks until you feel well enough to increase.

CFS - EB - Fibromyalgia
Attack RNA of muscle tissue.

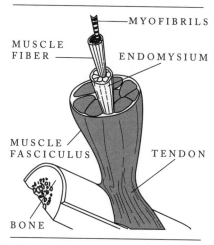

Associated connective tissues of the skeletal muscle.

In about six to eight weeks, it seems to break and you begin to rapidly get your life back. Usually you are pretty well fully recovered within six months, although it will take you longer to rebuild your immune system. Don't stop with the Liver and Immune until your CD4 count is back to high normal, near or at 1,200.

Something about this virus kills the body's ability to make xeronine, the alkaloid needed to repair cell walls and build the protein of the body. It used to take up to six months to get a person starting to get well, but once we added the Noni, a proxeronine that stimulates the production of xeronine, it sped up this recovery to a matter of about two months. Adding the VanChroZin, Platinum and Sulfur waters adds energy and strength, along with DHEA if you are over 40.

PRO-XERONINE
Stimulates the Body's
Ability to Make Xeronine

found in

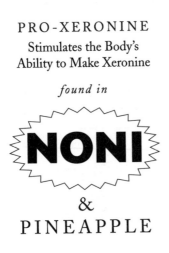

&
PINEAPPLE

XERONINE BONDS

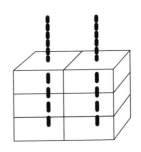

Protein consisting of polypeptides are held together by the alkaloid xeronine.

Chronic fatigue can also be caused from emotional roots such as feelings of rejection or feeling overwhelmed by circumstances you can't change. It seems that no matter what is causing their excessive tiredness, patients are being diagnosed as having chronic fatigue. It's another example of the medical profession's new fad, which is, "I don't know what is *really* wrong with you. Since I can't fix it with medicine, I'll just give your problem a name and hand you antidepressants."

CHRONIC SINUSITIS

This is either an allergy (weak immune system) or parasites. I suffered for years with sinus congestion, drainage and nasal itching as well as partial deafness in my right ear.

When I began to do a heavy parasite cleanse, my hearing gradually came back, but I still suffered from sinus problems and itching. I finally discovered tapeworm segments in my nasal passages and drainage from them. I have now gone back on the parasite cleanse with the Copper Solution, and the problem is clearing up. My sinuses are open for the first time in years.

CHROHN'S DISEASE

I believe that there is a severe food allergy that causes chronic diarrhea. If you have an allergy to anything, it works as a poison to the body, causing bloating, diarrhea, cramping, and irritated colon. The Intestinal Balancer helps control this until you get a chance to rebuild your immune system. I would highly recommend you do a parasite cleanse as I feel there could be a heavy infestation causing bowel problems. Because no one seems to address parasites, it is easily overlooked or misdiagnosed.

DIABETES

This is one disease that is definitely linked to a bad immune system. We are seeing juvenile diabetes (born with it or inherited) show up in families where it has never been present before. If you will look, you will find that many of these are being born to parents who got the polio shot or whose mothers are immune deficient. By the time he was 13, my nephew Christopher had been in and out of comas because of it. He couldn't eat any sweets or he would suffer. I put him on the Immune and Digestion (to stimulate the pancreas), and he has never suffered from another coma since. He can now even enjoy a piece of cake or sweets from time to time.

Onset diabetes usually comes from an immune system that is weakened due to age and environmental factors. As you control blood sugar with VanChroZinc, alpha lipoic acid, and diet, along with the blue program sheets, we usually find the need for insulin reduces and the degeneration in the heart and circulation reverses.

Please do not, I repeat, *DO NOT* GO OFF YOUR INSULIN until your doctor tells you to. It should be checked with blood and urine tests with doses regulated by your physician.

EMPHYSEMA AND CHRONIC BRONCHITIS

The lung consists of hundreds of little air sacs called alveolar that are lined with little hairs called cilia. The hairs move like a brush, cleaning out breathed-in debris, along with the fluids the body dumps through the lungs. It then eliminates all this by flushing these waste particles from our lungs as we exhale or cough. With pollutants like chemicals and cigarette smoke, the cilia are gradually killed and the alveolar walls gradually lose their elasticity. The pollution and dirt then remains in the lungs along with fluids from the lymph glands, and the person gradually drowns on their own waste and body fluids. They lose their ability to exchange air brought in by the lungs with the carbon dioxide from the blood, through the capillary walls. Thus the person becomes oxygen depleted throughout all the organs.

I have found that the Lung and Joint Formula helps quite a bit with this problem, as it contains expectorants to help clean the lungs a little bit, while it opens the lungs so it can exchange more oxygen/carbon dioxide.

Maile, who lives here in Oregon, has a brother with severe emphysema. He was house bound for quite some time, and couldn't go without oxygen supplementation. We started him on the Lung and Joint, and he immediately experienced relief. He was then able to occasionally go places without the constant need for oxygen as long as he took the capsules. One day, a friend of his who was selling products from another company talked him into using their product, claiming it was better than my Lung and Joint. In a very short time, he ended up in intensive care in the hospital, and not expected to live. His sister, Maile, came back and bought some more of the Lung and Joint and within two days, he was home again, doing well.

GOITER
This is easy to clear. All it takes is the Immune Formula and it gradually shrinks and disappears. Iodine is also beneficial.

GOUT
This is usually corrected with the Liver/Gallbladder and Immune formulas to clean out the blood and lymph glands (exercise helps, too, since it is the pump for the lymph glands). The Lung and Joint Formula also helps some.

HEPATITIS C
This is caused from the same Simian 40 retrovirus that attacks the cells of the liver. It can be cleared the same way we clear that retrovirus from any other part of the body: with the Four-Step Program mapped out on the blue sheets. The Liver/Gallbladder Formula has been successful in opening up the liver. Even when liver cancer is present, it causes the bilirubin to return to normal quite rapidly. The Herbal Extract seems to kill any form of virus, even the one that causes hepatitis A and hepatitis B.

HERPES

We have had a couple of herpes victims use the Herbal Extract with great success. This is very pervasive and takes longer to clear, but it can be done. I had a young man in Long Beach, California, contact me because he was going to be married and wanted to clear his system of herpes. He took the Herbal Extract for nearly a year, and the last time I talked to him, he was given a clean bill of health from his doctor.

LOU GEHRIG'S DISEASE

It is also called amyotrophic lateral sclerosis (ALS). With this disease, we have only been able to hold some of the symptoms and relieve others, but we are testing some new products we believe will help. One of these is Germanium, which is supposed to help restore the electrical impulses of the neurons. It is definitely improving memory in most people, too.

We have documentation of research linking this disease to the mercury fillings in the teeth. So the first thing you must do is remove all mercury from your mouth (don't remove more than two fillings a month as your system can't handle it), take alpha lipoic acid to chelate out the metals in your blood, and cleanse and rebuild the body.

If you look at the symptoms of ALS, you will see that they match perfectly the symptoms of mercury poisoning. If you examine Minamata Disease (mercury poisoning from eating fish from Japan's Minamata Bay, where mercury had been dumped), you will see the similarity of symptoms.

I have some outstanding films of TV documentaries of that incident, which show the victims in Minamata Bay. Many of them had the same symptoms as ALS sufferers (ALS only comes on a little slower). In the few cases I've dealt with, I have always found a lot of mercury fillings. Many of these clients had had their older fillings replaced with the newer ones—some of which were those that now contain 50 percent mercury, which is higher than it used to be.

Have you ever wondered why the dental profession has the highest rate of hair loss, divorce (caused from anger and irritability) and miscarriage, of any profession today? And doesn't it make you wonder why mercury, a known poison, must be handled as a toxic substance while dentists put it into your mouth?

Instruments are now available that measure the amount of mercury vapor that is released into our mouths while we chew. So be aware that, if you are a gum chewer, you are releasing high amounts of mercury vapor from your fillings into your mouth, lungs and body.

MULTIPLE SCLEROSIS

*Attacks RNA in the cells of connective tissue,
and the myelon sheath protecting spinal cord and nerves*

MULTIPLE SCLEROSIS
This one has been a very exciting adventure. We are seeing a GREAT DEAL OF SUCCESS with MS, but we do have to go slowly with the program. Again, we are dealing with the Simian 40 retrovirus that has attacked the connective tissue of the body, the myelon sheath on the spinal cord, and all the nerves. One of the most exciting responses has been the wonderful result we have had with the Sulfur Water. In just three days, the tremors stop and balance is restored.

Ida, who is a friend of mine, has suffered from this disease for twenty-five years. She had to drink with a straw, eat with a spoon, and wear a bib at meals because she shook so much. On only a tablespoon of Sulfur Solution each day, she is now able to hold a cup or glass of liquid, eat with a fork, and she doesn't need to wear a bib anymore. Her balance has greatly improved, her speech is much clearer, and she is even walking more.

I had used the Nerve and Muscle, which helped some. But when we added the Nerve and Muscle Plus, the numbness in Ida's feet vanished and much of the pain in her legs is going away. One of the other problems with this disease is terrible spasms. Ida has practically lived off Valium and other drugs, but nothing stopped them. When she feels a spasm starting, she takes a sip of the Calcium Water and, almost immediately, it stops. As she improves, we are adding more and more things, and hopefully we will win the battle.

Tish, who lives here in Oregon, is on the full program plus some of the waters. She has been experiencing the same response as Ida, and is now 95 percent improved and getting better and better all the time.

Beverly was diagnosed with MS several years ago. When I first met her, she had coordination problems, difficulty seeing, and other typical MS symptoms. She took the full program for about a year with nearly a complete recovery, except for her eyesight.

PARKINSON'S DISEASE

For Parkinson's, we use the full program plus Nerve and Muscle, Calmers (to help relieve stress), and Calcium, Sulfur (to stop tremors) Magnesium, Germanium, and Selenium waters. We have seen great improvement, but haven't worked with them long enough to see full recovery.

ROOT CANALS AND MERCURY FILLINGS

We have seen some wonderful books such as *The Root Canal Cover-Up* that explain the symptoms connected with this problem. Root canals are not recommended because it kills the nerve of a bad tooth but doesn't remove the tooth itself. Normally, the teeth move up and down in the jaw, pushing bacteria and other waste from the roots up into the mouth, where the waste is eliminated. But after root canals, the tooth no longer moves up and down, which allows the bacteria to remain in the jaw and seep down into the system to cause trouble. The teeth are also fed by hundreds of little vessels that go to all areas of the tooth. Since the root canal causes blockage in those vessels, bacteria have no place to get out, so it backs up in them, too, eventually seeping down into the body.

Different teeth can affect different areas of the body and cause diseases. For example, fillings or root canals in the molars can cause brain tumors and breast cancer; fillings and root canals in the teeth just behind the incisors can cause prostate cancer; and on it goes. Some of Hal Huggins' books will give you far more information than I can. There have been a lot of studies linking disease to this process. There are cases of some people who had gone blind and got their eyesight back when mercury was removed from their mouth.

There are many more diseases I have yet to deal with, but that will remain for the next book. In most of the cases above, I usually recommend that my clients use the blue sheet, which helps them stick to and keep track of where they are in the complete cleanse and rebuild program. In this chapter, we have dealt strictly with the physical body. I wish I could say that all our cases were as successful as those I have related, but that would be untrue. With God's help, and as our knowledge increases, the percentages of complete recoveries should also increase.

Now, let's try to understand some of the spiritual and emotional causes of illness.

SECTION III

Healing the Mind & Soul

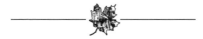

*I am come that they might have life,
and that they might
have it more abundantly.*

JOHN 10:10

Chapter 11

BOXING IN THE DARK

I n dealing with sick people, you must consider the whole person—body, soul and spirit. If you don't, it is like trying to hit your opponent in a boxing match in the dark. Sometimes you'll get in a lucky punch, but you will miss more often than you'll connect.

It's been proven that 85 percent of all illness has an emotional root. Dr. Bernie Siegel and others have written volumes about how the mind affects our physical health. We need to be very careful what we say to anyone with a potentially devastating disease. For many, just being told they have cancer means they'll accept it as a death sentence and immediately plan for their demise.

Health-care providers can use the same treatment on two people, and one will get well and the other will die. This is very frustrating to these providers who do everything they know of, physically and medically, and the patient still succumbs to the illness.

They are boxing in the dark.

But when you treat the whole person, it is like turning on the lights. At least now you know who or what your opponent is, which gives you a better chance of winning the battle.

I cannot emphasize enough the importance of searching out a good counselor or health-care provider who will address you as more than a body. It will facilitate your recovery and possibly save your life. If the caregiver will not address your emotional needs, rushes you through appointments with a quick exam, shoves pills at you without explaining what they do or their side affects, or treats you like a machine that pills will fix, then it is time to look for a new doctor.

Remember: YOU are paying the bill. It is YOUR BODY and yours alone that will suffer the consequences of what they do to you. So TAKE CONTROL of your circumstances and treatment. Go where they have time to see you as a WHOLE PERSON. What we think of ourselves greatly affects our health. You are a PERSON, EXTREMELY IMPORTANT to your family, to those who love you, and most of all, to GOD.

I can hear many of you saying, "Not me. No one would miss me if I weren't here. The world would be better off if I wasn't around." Let's see if that is really true and who, if anyone, would miss you.

How God Feels About You

First: He formed you—and since He doesn't make junk, you have a purpose.

Isaiah 44:2 says, "Thus says the Lord who made you and formed you from the womb, who will help you." Now, God was talking to the Nation of Israel, but since 2 Timothy affirms that "All Scripture is given by inspiration of God and is profitable for doctrine, for reproof, for correction, for instruction in right-eousness," it means that that applies to us, too. There are many, many more Scriptures to support this idea, but let's move on.

Second: You are so important to Him that He keeps a record of everything you've ever done or that has happened to you—and He is in control.

Matthew 10:29 states, "Are not two sparrows sold for a cop-per coin? And not one of them falls to the ground apart from your Father's will. But the very hairs of your head are all numbered." (Yes, guys, even those of you with only a few left!)

I can hear some of you ask, "If He loves me and knows so much about me, how come He placed me in that family that abused me?" Or "How come He allowed bad things to happen to me?" Well, we can't blame God for what people do. Read Jeremiah 29:11, "For I know the plans I have for you, plans to prosper you, not to harm you, plans to give you hope and a future." A lot of what happens to us is our own fault, born from poor judgment and headstrong attitudes that make us think we can do it on our own without first consulting Him.

In the Garden of Eden, God gave man a free will, and He doesn't violate that. I don't know all the answers, but I'm sure of one thing: Yesterday is gone. I can't change it, but He can make something good come out of it. Romans 8:28 tells us, "And we know that ALL things work together for good to those who love God, to those who are the called according to His purpose." We can let the past defeat us by sitting around harboring bitterness (letting it make us sick) or wallow in self-pity, or—as the above verse says—let *God* use it to make us a better, stronger person.

I believe the most important thing to our future are *not* the cards that life has dealt us, but what we *do* with them.

I love the old saying, "When life hands you lemons, make lemonade." Most of the great people of history are not ones who lived easy, wonderful, perfect lives. But they were the ones who made "lemonade." I also really appreciate Dr. Schuller's statement, "Tough times never last. Tough people do."

Third: God even knows our innermost thoughts and feelings.

Throughout Scripture, Jesus is called the Word of God. As we read Hebrews 4:12-13, we see that He even knows our innermost thoughts. Nothing—absolutely nothing—is hidden from Him. "For the Word of God is living and powerful, and sharper than any two-edged sword, piercing even to the division of soul and spirit, and of joints and marrow, and is a discerner of the thoughts and intents of the heart. And there is no creature hidden from His sight, but all things are naked and open to the eyes of Him to whom we must give account."

You know what is so amazing to me about this statement? How many people know you that well—or do you know that well—who would still be willing to die for the sake of the other? God did, for John 3:16 states, "For God so loved the world [and we're all a part of it] that He gave His only begotten Son, that whosoever believed in Him, will not perish, but have everlasting Life." That means all of us—including you.

Knowing us as He does, He still calls us His friend. John 15:13 tells us, "Greater love has no one than this, than to lay down one's life for his friends." It blows my mind that the Great God of the Universe calls me and you His friends!

Now I can hear many of you again asking, "Well then, why does He not stop all the bad things that are happening and just end it all?" There are several reasons. First, because friendship is a two-way street. You can't call people friends unless you both care about each other. He wants us to voluntarily love Him back. Second, because He has given us free will. Third, because He loves us so much.

Second Peter 3:9 says, "The Lord is long-suffering toward us, not willing that ANY [even you] should perish." He is giving us every chance in the book to accept His love and let Him come into our lives and change us so we can enjoy all the wonderful things He, in His great love for us, has prepared. John 14:2 assures us, "In my Father's house are many mansions, if it were not so, I would have told you. I go to prepare a place for you, and if I go and prepare a place for you, I will come again and receive you to Myself, that where I am, there you may be also."

Why would you want to spend eternity with Him if you don't even have time to spend one hour a week in church or spend time with His love letter to us, the Bible? Well, you won't, unless you get to know Him. Mankind is always looking to his own way of doing things or finding peace outside of a relationship with God. We suffer guilt that destroys us emotionally and physically, we lack peace in our innermost being because we are too proud to come to Him and ask His forgiveness for our sins. And we wonder why we are so sick?

Only God can heal the pain, frustrations, anger and guilt of our past and wipe them out completely. First John 1:9 tells us, "If we confess our sins, He is faithful and just to forgive us our sins and to cleanse us from all unrighteousness."

PHYSICAL HEALING STARTS WITH SPIRITUAL HEALING

If one looks at the statistics of anyone who has entered a drug-treatment center run by the medical profession or other groups that emphasize the physical aspect first, you will see that the rate of permanent cure is only about 3 percent. But if you look at Teen Challenge and other Christian-based centers that deal first with the person's *spiritual* side, *then* the drug problem, the rate of permanent cure is more than 90 percent—an astounding difference. Healing the body, without healing the soul first, is certainly boxing in the dark.

Matthew 25:41 tells us that hell was not made for man, but for Satan and his angels (demons). Satan knows he is doomed and where he is headed, so he is trying to take as many people as he can with him. As 1 Peter 5:8 warns, "Be sober, be vigilant; because your adversary the devil walks about like a roaring lion, seeking whom he may devour." And Matthew 10:28 admonishes us, "Do not fear those who kill the body [which includes anyone, even health-care providers] but cannot kill the soul. But rather fear Him who is able to destroy both body and soul in hell."

He knows you better than anybody else does. Yet He still loved you enough to choose to lay down His life for you. Now, that is love above anything another human being can give—and it is directed at *you*!

Romans 2:8 says, "For by grace you have been saved, by grace through faith, and that not of yourselves, it is the gift of God." Won't you begin your healing today and let Jesus come into your heart? He loves you so much. You cannot imagine the peace and joy that will be yours when you do.

OK, I can hear a lot of you say, "Yeah, maybe God loves me but nobody else would care if I wasn't here." Really? Try sitting down sometime and thinking back over your life to see what would have happened had you not been born. (Similar to what the angel showed George Bailey in "It's a Wonderful Life." George didn't think he'd be missed, either.)

What about your parents? Ask them if they feel you weren't important or if they wished you hadn't been born. Would they grieve if you died? In most cases, you bet they would! Don't project your depression on them, but see yourself from their point of view. Take an honest look at what they would experience, and maybe even sit down and talk to them. For you who are parents, I doubt that your children wish you had never been born, for then they wouldn't be here, either.

What about your spouse? Ask them if they think their life would have been happier or better without you. What about friends throughout your life? Would they have been happy to have never known you? What about animals you have loved or that have loved you? Do you think they would have been loved and cared for had you not been born?

BOXING IN THE DARK

Maybe you have never been married or haven't had children yet. Who knows what God has planned for you? Maybe you'll be the parent of the future president, world leader, or doctor who will find the cure for some "incurable" disease.

None of us are an island unto ourselves. We all impact the world and people around us in some way. I doubt that the parents of history's great people saw themselves as so remarkable that they deserved to produce great offspring.

I don't want to debate the abortion issue here, just make a simple comment. I'm sure glad my mother didn't believe in it, for I was the last of eight children, born to her when she was 45 years old. The last thing she wanted was another child, but she wouldn't abort me. I'd like to think that there are many others out there who are either enjoying their animals more or their good health because I was here to help.

OK, I just heard that. "Yeah, yeah, OK. So I'm important to God. I admit that there is *some* good come from my life because _____." (Just fill-in your own memory.) "But the world still wouldn't miss me. I'm not important; I'm just a lowly garbage man."

Just a lowly garbage man? Try running this world without you! Ask the hospital, the restaurants, the stores—ask *anybody*—if you aren't important. Each of us would be severely limited in our ability to do our jobs if we had to make frequent trips to the dump. And how many of us wouldn't go at all? Where would that leave us?

"OK, so I'm just a farmer." Just a farmer? Where would we all be if we had to grow our own food, milk cows (much less try to care for them in the city), grind wheat, bake bread, and on and on it goes.

No matter how small our job seems to be—or how insignificant we feel—somewhere we do, or will, make a difference in someone's life. Maybe someday we'll even save a life. So it's hard for me to believe that the world would have been better off had you never existed. Or better off if you left us now—whether by ending your life by suicide or by allowing sickness to do it for you.

Boy, I heard *that shout* all the way over here. You say that you're not allowing sickness to kill you, you just can't stop it? I'm afraid that all too many of you are allowing it, rather than facing the struggle of overcoming the inner problem that's causing the illness.

One classic example of this is a man called Worth, who lived in Portland, Oregon. I met him around 1994, when he came to me because of back and knee problems caused from so many years of kneeling as a roof layer. I started him on Nerve and Muscle, which gave him quite a bit of relief.

Through the years, we worked on rebuilding his liver and immune system. He often stopped to chat about politics and such. On the surface, I realized he had somewhat of a negative attitude, but in visiting his home, getting to know his lovely wife and children, all seemed pretty good until the spring of 1996.

Then I noticed that he began to lose a lot of weight and had some major changes in his complexion. He had been complaining of a lot of bowel problems, which we just couldn't get corrected. I have seen as many as ten cancer clients in a day, so I pretty well recognize when a person is suffering from it. He looked like a classic case to me, so I urged him to go to a doctor and get checked. He did, but all tests came back negative.

It was so baffling. Of all the people I know, this man had worked harder than anyone and taken nearly as much of my product as I had, and still he got sicker and sicker. If the average cancer client who uses my program had used as much as Worth did, they would have been well. But not Worth.

The mystery began to unveil as the sicker he became, the more his true feelings began to show—feelings that many of us couldn't believe this sweet old man harbored. Bottled up inside him was a caldron of hatred and rage that had spilled out on everyone in his life. He had abused his wife and children unmercifully for all their lives. It all stemmed from his hatred for his mother and his contempt for his father for not standing up for Worth when he was small. When it came to light it became all too apparent why the cancer had struck his bowels and bladder. He couldn't and wouldn't eliminate the anger, so it destroyed the elimination canals of his body.

When a doctor finally found the cancer, he was in real trouble. In spite of all our herbs, he got worse and worse. I pled with him to deal with the anger and rage or it would kill him, but he just couldn't. All his life, it had been such an all-consuming part of him that he just wouldn't face it and let it go. He said he had accepted Christ as his Savior, but he wouldn't give his rage to God so He could heal the little boy inside.

Worth knew his rage was killing him. But he tried to deal with it by not getting angry anymore, not letting anyone around him say or do anything to make him mad. Everyone had to walk on eggshells around him, but he could never "see" that the way to deal with it was to get the rage and anger out of his heart. It had to start with him, not others around him. Because he refused to deal with his heart and emotion, it killed him. He preferred to die—and did die—rather than face the heart change he needed in order to live.

Unfortunately, I have seen this pattern all to often. For some reason, the mind is more willing to stay in the familiar patterns we have established for it. It takes a lot of courage and strength to break out. The fear of facing what caused the problem becomes bigger and bigger in our lives until it becomes an insurmountable barrier. Fear is like that. The more we think about it, the bigger and bigger it gets until the fear itself is bigger than the thing we are afraid of.

Most of the time, if we can find the courage to take an honest look at the problem and deal with it, we find out the real problem wasn't so big after all. Sometimes it takes professional help to get us to that point. So if your life is important enough to you and to others (it already is to God), then you may need to pursue that avenue with a good psychologist or minister.

Satan will keep you bound in your fears as long as he can. But you've given that problem a stronghold in your life long enough. Hasn't it taken enough from you yet or caused you enough pain? Don't let it rob from you anymore. Break those chains that are destroying you!

WHAT CAN I DO NOW TO CORRECT THE MESS I'M IN?

First: Get spiritually right with God to attain peace of mind and freedom from the past. Only He can do that. Yesterday is gone. You can't change it, but you can change the future and get rid of the feelings and attitudes that are making you sick, crippling you, and keeping you from experiencing a better life.

Second: Realize that we are all born equal in God's eyes. Since God is no respecter of persons, then there is no limit to what He can do through a life given over to Him.

Years ago, when I first started doing television, my bad self-image made it hard for me to believe that God could use me and make something good of my life. One day I met Roy Rogers and Dale Evans, my childhood heroes. They were sweet, shy, humble, loving people who struck me as just ordinary folks who had given their lives to God and allowed Him to guide and use them. They often sang the popular song, "It is no secret what God can do, what He's done for others, He'll do for you. With arms wide open, He'll pardon you, it is no secret, what God can do."

It was like a light went on in my head, and I heard, *Give me your life and you will be surprised what I can make of it.*

I asked back, "Why me, Lord?"

His response was as clear as if I'd heard an audible voice. *Why not? You are no different than any of my other children, and if you let me lead you, I'll prove it.*

Why not? You are no different than any of My other children, and if you let Me lead you, I'll prove it. Until that point in my life, I had considered myself as being one big screw up, making one bad decision after another. I knew I could never change things or be any better unless God did something. That meeting changed my life forever.

Third: Ask God for wisdom. The dictionary defines wisdom as "the power or faculty of forming a sound judgment in any matter; having the power of discerning and judging rightly."

How do I accomplish the things I relate in this book, and where did I get the wisdom contained in it? One place: from God.

When I was growing up, I used to wonder what I would be as an adult and how I would make a good living or find the right man to marry? Where can I make the most money to have the *things* I wanted? This was important to me, as I am sure it is to many of you, especially since we were struggling, fairly poor people. One day I read some verses in Proverbs 8 that showed me I had the cart in front of the horse:

Wisdom is better than rubies, and all the things one may desire cannot be compared with her. I, wisdom, dwell with prudence and find out knowledge and discretion. By me kings reign, and the judges of the earth. I love those who love me, and those who seek me diligently will find me. Riches and honor are with me, enduring riches and righteousness. My fruit is better than gold, yes, than fine gold and my revenue than choice silver. I traverse the way of righteousness in the midst of the paths of justice, that I may cause those who love me to inherit wealth, that I may fill their treasures.

From that day on, I was determined to seek knowledge and wisdom. If I had that, then I knew I would have all the other things I needed in life. James 1:5 states, "If any of you [means just what it says with no discrimination] lacks wisdom, let him ask of God, who gives to ALL liberally and without reproach, and it will be given to him" (or her). No qualifications to fill *first*, just ask Him.

I had been aware of this in my youth and pursued it, for a time, but lost sight of it in my mid-20s—until that meeting with Dale and Roy. I had lost my way for awhile, but I now knew that God could turn it around and make something good come out of it. I now sought wisdom and His will with all my heart. It still was not a perfect walk, but it was the beginning of some real growth in my life.

Since you are no different from any other person God has created, then He can work His miracle in you, too.

Finally—Learn to trust God. Remember, anyone who loves you as much as He does is definitely someone you can trust to do and give you the best there is.

He formed you. He came to earth specifically to die for you that your sins could be forgiven and you could become His friend. He has gone back to Heaven to prepare a mansion for you. He is patient and long-suffering, waiting for you to come to Him so He can begin the rebuilding process in your life.

"Eye hath not seen, nor ear heard, nor have entered into the heart of man, the things which God has prepared for those who love Him" (1 Corinthians 2:9).

"For I know the plans I have for you, plans to prosper you, not to harm you, plans to give you hope and a future" (Jeremiah 29:11).

Now *that's* someone you can trust.

Chapter 12

BLIND SPOTS

W hat is a blind spot? It's a concept, a fear, an idea or an action that causes us problems, either emotionally or socially, and blocks the achievement of our goals. We may or may not "see" it, but the longer it is there, the bigger it looms and the harder it is to "face it" and let it go.

Sometimes, it is something that happened to us when we were small that became embedded in our minds, and affects the way we see things relating to it now. We become comfortable in what we know, whether it is painful or not, and it takes courage to break past the barriers in our mind. But once we do, we find out it wasn't so bad, and the problem is dispelled.

I touched on this in the last chapter, but it is so important, I feel I need to address it from another aspect. I don't think that blind spots are usually as serious and life threatening as what we have already covered. But they can be very devastating and, possibly, deadly.

This chapter is best explained by using a lot of examples.

As long as I can remember, I was terrified of dead bodies. I always had a picture in my mind that they were going to sit up and come after me if I went near them. When I was a college student, I worked as a nurse's aid at the local hospital. One night, there was a man who was dying and the staff, being busy, didn't want to leave him alone, so they told me to go in and sit with him until he was dead. I was absolutely terrified to be in that room alone with someone who might soon be a corpse.

I sat by the door and, when I thought he was dead, I rushed out to tell the nurse. When they checked him, he was not. They made me stay with him until I checked his pulse to be sure he was gone and said to me, "Don't leave again until he is definitely deceased." I have never spent a longer, more frightening night in all my life as I sat glued by that door.

When they finally pronounced him dead, they told me to give him a bath before he was sent downstairs. There was no way in the world I would have been able to do that. Thank God, they understood and didn't force me. Yet no one, at that time, really understood *why* I felt that way.

There was no way you could get me near a cemetery or any spot on the road where a person or animal had been killed, so we always went out of our way to avoid it. I knew they were going to rise up out of the grave or suddenly appear where they had been killed and come after me.

Now, I am a person with a strong faith in God, and although I couldn't see any logical reason for my fear, I ran from it most of my life. Finally, through counseling, it came out that when I was about 5 years old my brothers had taken me to see a Zombie movie in which bodies rose from their graves and stalked the villagers. Knowing the source of the fears didn't lessen them, until my brother died and I determined with my will to touch him. I went in alone to see his body, fighting my fear and breaking the hold it had on my life.

Yes, I have finally conquered that fear, but there is still a residue that makes me uncomfortable around bodies and graves. Most of it is dispelled, though, and I am no longer bothered by cemeteries, bodies or places where people or animals died. I am sure glad because now I'm able to be part of a search-

and-rescue team that must often deal with bodies. Thank God that this problem was dealt with *early enough* for me to go on with my life.

But the next one wasn't.

All my life, I believed that men did not love, were self-serving, and put their desires above those of their families. I had seen, on the surface, what looked like love from men. But in my heart I just couldn't believe they had the capacity to love. No amount of talking or reading to the contrary could change my attitude, and I was always puzzled as to why I felt that way.

Later in life, I would find out that this attitude was tied to my infertility. I love children and always have. I wanted to be married and have a family so badly I could taste it. When I was married, I became pregnant four times, but always lost the baby during the early part of the fourth month. I hounded doctors to find out why I couldn't carry them to term, but they could never find anything physically wrong. Unfortunately, they were boxing in the dark, and we didn't know it.

The counselor couldn't find any reason for the miscarriages either, except that perhaps my body was rejecting the baby because of the bad, abusive marriage I was living in at the time.

If you have ever experienced a miscarriage, you know how painful it is. After my divorce, I knew that my biological clock was running down, so I made a last ditch effort by trying artificial insemination at a fertility clinic. I was overjoyed when I became pregnant, and somehow knew I was carrying a blond-haired, blue-eyed boy.

I thought that surely this one would make it because I was no longer dealing with the abuse and stress of my marriage. But my world came crashing down when in the fourth month, my body again aborted.

There was something more that I just couldn't put my finger on. For ten years after that, I couldn't be around newborn babies without crying. Whenever they had a baby dedication at church, I had to leave until it was over.

Why had God done this to me, and why couldn't men love? When it was too late to have a child, I finally stopped long enough to find out what had happened. It wasn't God, but something that happened when I was in my fourth month in my mother's womb.

I'm sure you are asking how I found out. Well, it was by using the same techniques that I had used in communicating with the animals—except this time, I went back into my own memory. One thing that clued me into doing this was a book called *The Making of a Genius.* In this book, a couple read to their baby, talked to her, played classical music for her—before she was born. After her birth, the baby learned at a phenomenal speed, loved classical music, and graduated from college as a teenager. She was classified as a genius, but they were able to prove that what she received as a fetus also developed in her as she grew up.

As I traveled back through my memory, all the way back to birth, my attitude about men still existed in my mind. I then went back into my mind to my prenatal stage, and I found it, at the beginning of my fourth month of existence. Now this may seem a bit bizarre, for I didn't believe that a baby this early in development could "understand" or be "programmed," or that the brain developed enough to absorb anything. It was supposed to be a nonliving fetus—yet I heard something as clearly as though I were an adult listening to my mother talk.

When my mother, a tired 45-year-old woman who had already raised seven children, learned she was pregnant with me, she exclaimed, "Oh no! Not another child. I can't take any-more responsibility! That sexist husband of mine doesn't care about anything but satisfying his own desires. He doesn't care what it does to me."

I was floored. I spoke with my sister who confirmed my sus-picions, as she had been there when Mom said it. All those years, I had lived with an attitude programmed into me at the beginning of my fourth month of existence—an attitude that caused me a lifetime of pain and an empty home without the children I longed for. It wasn't life threatening, but it *was* heart-breaking.

Finally, I was able to "see" that men can love, too, when I was able to get rid of the mental block that said, "No they can't." If this can happen in a godly home, with a solid background, is it no wonder we have so many problems in this generation with so many children being born to teenagers and unwed mothers? Or being born into marriages in conflict in which pregnant women are abused or use drugs and alcohol?

A former animal-communication student of mine, Dorothy, related an experience she had during her third month of pregnancy. She is very good at communicating with animals, so her mental sensitivity was greater than just her emotions. She, being an unwed mother with a little girl to care for, decid-ed to have an abortion with her second pregnancy. She sud-denly felt an overwhelming grief and fear, and the baby became very active. It was so devastating to her that she couldn't go through with terminating her pregnancy. I am sure the baby knew what was going on and let her know he didn't want to die.

The reality of what the fetus feels was also brought home to me while working with a child psychologist in San Diego, California. Occasionally he would have a difficult case he couldn't figure out, especially if the child was very small or couldn't verbalize his or her feelings.

He brought a 5-year-old girl to me who had been adopted when she was a little younger than a year old. But now the marriage of the adoptive couple was dissolving. The girl was very angry and combative toward her adoptive mother, but clung to her father. The therapist could not figure out why because the adoptive mother had loved the girl very much and had only given her a loving, solid home until now.

I went back in the child's memory until I found the problem. She had been born to a teenager whose pregnancy had been an emotional roller coaster but who wanted to keep her baby. She went to school and held down a job while trying to care for her baby, but she couldn't afford childcare and didn't have family that would help. So while she went to work, she left the baby for hours in a crib with a bottle. Things were bearable for awhile, but the pressures of the load she carried became too much for her young mind. So she finally rejected the baby, giving it up for adoption.

Now, the child sensed the imminent breakup and subconsciously feared that her adoptive mother would also reject and leave her. Since she had no father in her early infancy, the father's leaving was no threat. So she struck out at the mother, testing whether she would keep her or not. But what she was really expressing was her anger toward her birth mother for her neglect and rejection.

The psychologist then began to treat her real problem. The last I heard, they planned to work toward the adoptive mother keeping her, while also working through the child's anger, reassuring her that this mom loved her and would be there for her. Had they not been able to find the child's real problem and work toward a resolution, this would have affected her relationships for the rest of her life—creating a blind spot that no one would have understood.

Another case I worked on was Andy, in Hamilton, Ohio. When I first met Andy, he was two years old, diagnosed as autistic, and was unable to sleep. From the time he was born, he was a relaxed, sweet, unresponsive baby, except when he would start to fall asleep. Then, he would begin screaming and tighten up into a ball. So they felt they had to give him drugs to relax him and put him to sleep. The only way they could get him to eat was by forcing food down his throat until his automatic swallowing reflex caused him to swallow. He had never given any indication that he recognized his father, and had been unresponsive to any teaching from his mother.

When I went back into his memory, I found him to be a happy, contented baby in the womb. But as I began to relive the birth experience, suddenly I began to choke, to the point where I nearly passed out. His mother did confirm that Andy had indeed been choked by the umbilical cord during the birth process. They just assumed that his problems had come from oxygen depravation, but I learned from him that he had mentally blocked out the birth experience. As far as he was concerned, it was too traumatic for his infant mind to deal with, so he had withdrawn to prenatal existence. As a fetus, you don't have to swallow, so he didn't. Every time he started to fall asleep, he began to relive the choking experience, making him scream in fear.

–I had been reading some books by Ruth Carter Stapelton, *The Gift of Inner Healing* and *The Experience of Inner Healing*. In her books, she talks about our mental blocks due to trauma and how they keep us from experiencing our full potential. She also gives techniques of visualization, of going back in our memory to an incident and *changing* our memory of that incident to lessen our related trauma. I decided to try some of these techniques with Andy to see if we could work him through the birth trauma. Since he was, in reality, mentally only a prenatal infant, I decided to use that particular technique for him.

I took Andy in my arms and began the process. I literally imagined myself as him, in the womb. I could feel the excitement at the beginning of the birth process until we got to the part when I could feel the cord touch "my" throat. Until that point, Andy had been relaxed, but as the cord touched my throat, Andy began to scream and tighten into a ball.

Next, I visualized the cord breaking and the birth being normal, with his mom and dad cuddling and loving him. Then he began to relax and look around. I then instructed his mom to do some of the techniques with him. In a prone position, she laid him on her abdomen. She visualized him as prenatal, projecting to him how much she wanted him and how excited she was that he was coming. She went through the same exercise I did, with the same response from Andy.

After we finished, Andy was very relaxed, and in a matter of only a few minutes, he fell into a deep sleep, WITHOUT DRUGS. I asked his mom to let me know what would happen with Andy, and was thrilled to hear from her a couple days later. She reported that Andy had slept almost constantly for the next twenty-four hours, again without sleeping drugs. Why not? He was exhausted because sleep *without* drugs is the only true, restful sleep.

As Andy began to "wake up" from his condition, he began asking for his bottle and started crawling. When his dad would come home from work, Andy crawled right to him and indicated he wanted to be picked up. He began to rapidly progress through the post-birth stages, but as the drugs began to leave his system he started going through withdrawal.

I had warned his mother to watch out for that because I knew he'd be addicted after two years of having drugs. Sure enough, he became fussy, had diarrhea, and exhibited all the normal symptoms of drug withdrawal, even though he continued responding to people and his environment. Yet his mother panicked and took him back to the doctor.

Now remember, he had been on drugs for two years, and had now only been off them for five days. The doctors couldn't admit he had been addicted or that we had helped Andy at all. His was now a totally different pattern of behavior not connected to falling asleep. Instead, he acted the way a child would act when sick with the flu or from teething—or when going through drug withdrawal. But they immediately put Andy back on drugs, and the last I could learn was that he was again doped up and regressing.

What a sad thing to make those tremendous strides—then revert back because of the medical profession's pride. They just couldn't admit that Andy had been addicted to drugs and had been helped by something *other* than those drugs. This child's life will never reach the potential God designed it to. His parents will never know the joys of watching him grow up normally, which was their right to do.

Sometimes it is so hard, even impossible, to get past the programming we have had all our lives in which we're taught that whatever the doctor says *is law* and there is no other way. There are some good doctors who understand what we did. Unfortunately, Andy's were not among them.

Another time I was working with a group of rodeo-horse people in the Fresno, California area when I met Betty. We began to talk about how she felt that things in her life just weren't right. Her husband, the love of her life, had been electrocuted on the job while replacing electrical lines that were thought to be dead. She seemed to be able to handle it to some degree, and even went on to remarry. But she could never let go of her first husband. She dreamed about him, thought of him all the time, and even had difficulty relating to her present husband or letting him make love to her. She felt unfaithful while outwardly was going on with her life.

The more she talked, the more suspicious I became about his death. In her mind, he was not dead. When I asked her if she had ever seen him in the casket, she said no, just as I had suspected. The last time she had seen him was the morning he left for work, when he kissed her good-bye and said, "I'll see you tonight." But he never came home, and in her mind, he was out there somewhere. I knew that until she "saw" him dead, she could not accept it.

This is probably the hardest thing anyone has to face when a loved one disappears. Even if you *mentally* believe they are dead or are told they are dead—until you have a body to see and bury, and know *beyond a shadow of a doubt* in your heart and mind, that they are truly gone—they can still be alive to you. Maybe someone made a mistake, you might tell yourself, and that coffin doesn't *really* contain my loved one.

Betty's blind spot was refusing to look at her beloved's body and accept his death. It was keeping her from going on with the present and relating to the wonderful man she now called her husband. No matter how hard her husband tried, he couldn't change her heart.

Well, I asked Betty if she was ready to work through the trauma. It had stolen several years from her relationship, and she admitted that she now needed and wanted to go on, but didn't know how. I warned her it would be emotionally painful, but she would have to work through the pain she should have worked through at the funeral. She was willing.

We sat down together and she closed her eyes. I led her through that last day, the breakfast, the good-bye kiss, his wave to her as he walked away, and his loving, wonderful smile. We then moved up to the phone call and the events of the day when she was told of his death. I had her picture Jesus standing there, holding her up with His loving arms around her, as she heard the news.

We then continued to the morgue, still with Jesus holding her close. I told her to look at the body on the table. She said she could see it, but it was covered up with a sheet. I told her to mentally pull the sheet back and look at her husband. She kept saying, "I can't, I can't," while I gently urged her on until she was finally able to pull back the sheet in her mind.

At this point, she began to cry. With each breath she took, her heart-wrenching sobs became more and more intense. She cried and cried until she was able to talk again. Then we worked through the rest of the funeral—which had an open casket this time. Again she kissed her husband good-bye, but next she experienced the lonely, empty days that followed. This time, we made sure that each of her pictures also had Jesus holding her and quietly weeping with her.

You may wonder why be so cruel and put her through that heartache? I knew that until she "saw" him, whether in reality (which was impossible at this stage), or in her mind, his death had to become real. She had to say good-bye or she would never be able to go on with tomorrow. She was emotionally drained and didn't have a tear left, but she did express a tremendous release.

The last I heard, she was growing in her relationship with her present husband and she was now able to totally live in the present, enjoying the blessing God has given her. Her first husband is now a fond, wonderful memory.

197

I began to apply some of the healing of memories to my own life, and they worked. I had always grown up thinking that I was never good enough to succeed. In this second chapter, I related my experience with a grade-school teacher and the pain success brought to my young mind. I knew that in order to succeed in my adult life and be able to do television successfully, I needed to change my memories about trying and succeeding. In the past, whenever I was just about to attain a goal or succeed, I would subconsciously jeopardize what I had set out to do. I always failed, which reinforced my feeling that I was a failure and just couldn't do it.

I remember once when I had a part in a high-school play. All I had to do was stand there, smile and say (I'll never forget those three words) "I like boys." I was so scared. Now I don't remember anything else about that play, except that I couldn't get those words out no matter how hard I tried. The prompter had to whisper them over and over until I finally blurted them out.

Since I'd read Ruth Carter Stapelton's book (she is President Carter's sister and her husband is a retired veterinarian), I began to go back through all the memories I could recall where I had failed. I pictured Jesus with me, and visualized success instead of what really happened. I built new memories to replace old ones. Gradually I began to daydream about being on television and being so popular that I even won awards. I pictured people asking for my autograph, telling me how wonderful I was, clapping for me, and on and on it went

Gradually, I began to believe that I could succeed. When the opportunity did arrive for me to appear on some shows, they were *very* popular and successful. No, I never won any awards, but I did accomplish what I set out to do: break the pattern of failure and replace it with patterns of success. It worked and I am grateful. Television was not the fear I had felt in high school, but was and continues to be, a lot of fun. I have no problems standing in front of a crowd, either. Now I love it.

I had a friend, whom I will call Jim, who has a blind spot he refuses to see and deal with. When I first met him at church, we hit it off beautifully. For six months we spent all our free time together. At first he was loving and affectionate, but suddenly he withdrew physically. I didn't think too much of it because we just enjoyed being together and doing things. I really felt he had developed a love for me as I had grown to feel for him. But to my regret and deep heartache, I would learn that he had a blind spot that he was, and still is, not willing to release.

When I was preparing to return to California, where I lived, he just flat out told me he could never love me because I wasn't physically attractive to him. He had an image of what he wanted in a woman, and he would settle for nothing less. She had to be tiny, flat-chested, much younger than him, and pretty, much like a ballerina. Since I am physically just the opposite, and I couldn't change my physical attributes, I left. I never intended to fall in love with him or anyone, but I did, and carried a broken heart for eight years. I know he cared deeply for me because of things he said and did. We balanced each other beautifully, but he couldn't get past the blind spot of his image.

We remained friends for about thirteen years. I watched him pray that God would send Him a wife and, at age 47, his "fantasy" came into his life. She was pretty, short, flat-chested and skinny. It did no good for anyone to talk with him to help him see that his "image" could have an accident tomorrow and be changed forever in her looks, that it is the *person* that is important. He was in love with an image, a dream, and he just couldn't "see" what any of us were saying. He was sure she was sent by God, and he had to have her. He was deeply in love.

The next thing I heard, he was married. Much to my sorrow, what we predicted came true. He found out his fantasy had feet of clay and, as problems developed, he left her. Within one year, they divorced. It is so sad, because he is a wonderful person with great potential, but he will never attain it until he lets go of his blind spot.

Many times, during our long friendship, we have talked about his first marriage. Jim tried to blame the marriage problems on her, but I observed something a little different, which would make any woman look elsewhere for acceptance. She had been thin and pretty when they married, but she had gained some weight and developed a tummy after their son was born. Knowing Jim the way I do, I know he kept reminding her of how she looked (even though she was only about a size 10 with a tummy most of us would be happy to have).

When I tried to bring this up, he'd get angry and deny he'd ever say those things. Yet EVERY TIME he saw her, when I was around, the first comment out of his mouth was about her gaining weight. She had wanted to get back together, but by this time she had gained quite a bit of weight, and he would have no part of it. They had other problems, yet I'm sure he believes that these other problems were their *only* problems because he refuses to admit when he's at fault (another blind spot) or that he can't accept her because she is heavier.

He became very angry when I mentioned this to him just a few years ago when we went to pick up his son at her home. He told me to never bring it up again because he didn't do that anymore. Yet when we walked into the house, his first words were, "Gee, Susie, you sure have put on more weight, haven't you?" Sad to say in his case, as with most people who refuse to deal with their blind spots, he became very angry and denied what he was actually saying. Even if I had had a tape recorder and proved it to him, he still would have denied it until he was ready to face the truth.

A couple years ago, I told Jim that if he didn't grow up and get the little-girl look out of his fantasy, he will be 75 years old and still praying that God would bring him the perfect woman. I believe that even more now, for long after his fantasy blew up in his face, he still blames her for their problems and refuses to face that he chose a fantasy and not a real woman.

The last I've heard, he was pursuing another girl who was just like the last one (remarkably, she also had the same last name). My heart breaks for him because he just won't get beyond his fantasy to find and experience the great potential God chose for him.

When I grew up, I never saw my father lay a hand on my mother, except with love. I always thought that marriage was sacred, for I had always seen my dad exhibit nothing but fidelity.

One time, my brother sent my dad to a house to bid on replacing a roof (they worked together as carpenters), only to find my dad walking down the street, mad as a hornet. When my brother asked him what was wrong and about the bid, my dad blurted out, "That hussy! She came to the door and asked me to come in and she was buck naked. How dare she act like that!" He had responded to her invitation by quickly turning and walking away.

Now don't get me wrong, my dad was no saint. But he was a godly, moral, honest man who lived those principles before us kids, and I will always love him for that. When I got married, I expected my husband, who said he loved me, to be the same.

What a surprise I got when, one month after we were married, my husband started cheating on me and beating me.

Sometimes he beat me so badly that I couldn't go out for a week because I had black-and-blue marks all over me.

Because I didn't believe in divorce, I lived with that for nine years. Every time I went for counseling, I was told that it was all my fault. It was always the woman's fault for if I would try harder, then I could please him and he wouldn't beat me. My husband also told me that if I pleased him and did what he wanted, then he would love me. But if I didn't, he wasn't obligated to love me. So every night, the house was so clean you could eat off my floors, dinner was on the table, his bath was drawn and his clothes, laid out. Then I'd think that, *surely*, I must have pleased him this time, and he would love me.

But then he would put on a white glove and check the baseboards for dust or point out steam from his bath water on the bathroom mirror—all the while complaining about the bad deal he got with such a filthy wife. After all, he'd say, he had to go to work all day and support this mess. Since I was so lazy, why didn't I go out and get a job so I'd have something to do?

So I did. Yet when I went to work, he complained that it made him look bad as a husband that he couldn't provide for his wife. So I eventually quit, only to find out he had taken all the money I'd earned and spent it on himself and his mother, in Europe. He would then find things to complain about until he felt justified to go out drinking all night, leaving me alone to cry for hours.

The marriage became such a nightmare that one day, as I was driving, I suddenly "came to" and realized I was heading straight toward a telephone pole at about 60 miles per hour to kill myself. After that, I committed myself to a mental hospital because I thought something was wrong with me that I couldn't be a good wife and please my husband.

For years, I was beaten, got concussions from having my head pounded against walls, and lived through hell. My situation finally came to a head when one night he chased me into a field and tried to kill me by wrapping barbed wire around my neck. How I escaped is still a blur.

The next day, after he went to work, I packed my car with my personal belongings, took my dogs, and left. I never went back. It was one of the biggest heartbreaks of my life. After my divorce, it took years of healing and the loving support and care of Pastor Jack Hayford before I was able to pick up the pieces and build a new life.

Now, I can hear you say, what was all *that* for? What does that have to do with the cost of tea in China? Is she trying to evoke sympathy or something? No dear friend, I only wanted you to see that sometimes we develop blind spots that have a legitimate root, but unless we let God heal us, it will destroy His best for our future.

Although I loved being married and having a home, my marriage had left some pretty deep scars. It wasn't until I reached 58 years of age that I realized I had let the experiences of my past create a blind spot in me. I was so terrified of marriage that every time I met someone I cared about, I subconsciously jeopardized that relationship, or my mind would become constantly flooded with all his faults and every small reason—real or imagined—why it could never work.

I always went for men that I knew I'd never marry, or who wouldn't be interested in me, because I really couldn't face marriage with *anyone*. I have had some pretty special men in my life who would have made good husbands and fathers (and did!). But I just couldn't get past my blind spot. I couldn't let go of my hurts and let God heal me, so I could enjoy the blessings He so wanted to give me

There were times I did this with Jim, too—and look at the pain I needlessly suffered because of it.

One day, I stopped by my former husband's shop to get something and found out he had been happily married to another woman for over twelve years (I wonder if she'd describe her marriage as happy, too). It suddenly dawned on me that he had gone on with his life, but I had continued to carry the wounds that prevented me from going on with mine. I had continued to allow him and Satan to rob me of a marriage and family—not only back then, but for the twenty-five years that followed.

As I left his shop that day, I decided that they had *both* had enough of my life, and they weren't getting any more. With God's help, I finally faced my blind spot of fear and Satan's lie that all men are self-serving, self-centered and abusive.

No, I am not remarried nor am I currently interested in anyone. But at last I'm free to love again and build a home, should God so choose. I am glad that God doesn't have only "Plan A" for our lives, but that in His love and mercy, He does have back-up plans in case we miss His best.

If I've learned anything in my 59 years, it is to trust God, to ask Him about *everything* before jumping in, and to face my blind spots before they can take away years of my life.

I wish I could say that I have totally arrived, but I can't. But we—God and I—are working on it. I am so grateful that I serve a loving Father who is incredibly patient. He only weeds out one problem at time. Like growing up, it happens in stages. We don't go from infancy to maturity in a few short months.

If you are earnestly seeking God's best for you, He will weed out your blind spots, one at a time, IF YOU WILL LET HIM. That's the key. He will never force His best on us, but if you come to Him and ask, He'll do it.

Weeding out those blind spots is no picnic. It can be painful, but like a diseased or infected part of the body, it has to be removed or it will infect the whole body and keep you from attaining your physical best. A blind spot will hinder your full development and rob you of the great joy God has intended for you.

Just remember, if you don't let go of your old hurts, it is *you* who will continue to suffer—not the ones who hurt you. It is you who will remain scarred with unresolved pain, anger and bitterness. It's likely that the one who brought this pain will have already gone on with his or her life—without giving you a second thought.

My ex-husband taught me that. As I left his shop that day, he jokingly asked me why I had never remarried. I flipped back, "My first marriage was enough. It was too traumatic and painful to want to try again." He honestly looked puzzled and quietly said, "Hey, *I* was that marriage." I replied, "You got it." To this day, I don't believe he even knows what he did, but I have allowed it to rob me.

What is your blind spot? How long will you let it keep you from enjoying a full, healthy, abundant life? Won't you let God help you remove it? Just savor His promises in the following verses:

"I am come that they may have life, and that they may have it more abundantly" (John 10:10).

"These things I have spoken to you, that My joy may remain in you, and that your joy may be full" (John 15:11).

"Now may the God of hope fill you with all joy and peace in believing, that you may abound in hope by the power of the Holy Spirit" (Romans 15:13).

And do you know what is the best part of all? You don't have to face it alone. He will be with you, giving you courage, strength and comfort, because He longs to see you free to enjoy all the good things He has planned for you.

Right in front of my chair where I sit for my daily devotions is a bulletin board where I keep certain items and pictures of people I want to remember in prayer. In the center is a plaque that I love because it reminds me of WHO is walking with me today. The plaque reads:

> *"Lord, help me to remember that nothing is going to happen to me today that You and I together can't handle."*

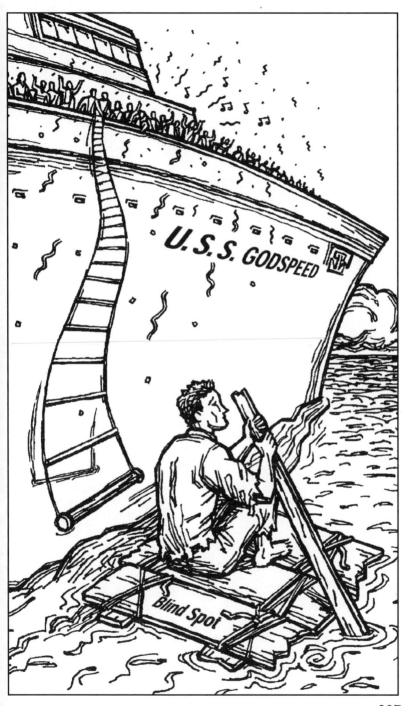

Chapter 13

SUICIDE:
The Ultimate Blind Spot

And ye shall know the TRUTH,
and the TRUTH shall make you free.

JOHN 8:32

I am the way,
the TRUTH, and the life.

JOHN 14:6

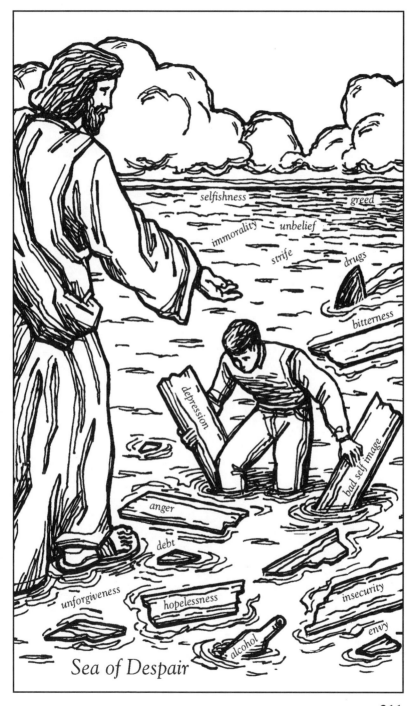

Chapter 14

ANGELS

I include this chapter with the hope that it will encourage you to trust God to a greater extent, knowing that He watches over you and is prepared to send His ministering angels should you need them.

In recent years, volumes have been written about angels and how they intervene in our lives. Throughout my life, God has sent them to rescue me many times, proving over and over His wonderful concern for my welfare. Some of them I have seen and some I have not, but I knew they were there. I felt them and "saw" the results, much like one can't see the wind, but can feel it and see its affect.

Satan may be about, seeking whom he may devour, but God is stronger than he is. In fact, if you read the account of Job, you will learn that he can't even touch the child of God without God's permission. First John 4:4 states, "You are of God, little children, and have overcome them, because He [the Holy Spirit] who is in you is greater than he who is in the world [Satan and his angels, the demons].

But wait, you say. Aren't we all of God? No, we are not, and those who aren't are much more open to the attack and possession of Satan and his demons than the child of God. Even Jesus told the religious leaders of His day that although they devoted their lives to "religion," they still didn't know Him, the One who religion is supposed to be all about.

John 8:44,47 declares, "You are of your father the devil, and the desires of your father you want to do. He was a murderer from the beginning and does not stand in the truth because there is no truth in him. When he speaks a lie, he speaks from his own resources, for he is a liar and the father of it. He who is of God hears God's words; therefore you do not hear because you are not of God."

We aren't all children of God, as the New Agers would like you to believe. Romans 3:23 tells us that "All have sinned and come short of the glory of God." And Romans 5:8 says, "But God demonstrates His own love toward us, in that while we were still sinners, Christ died for us."

Before Christ came, man's sins were forgiven as he brought animals, without any blemish, to the temple. They laid their hands on the animal symbolizing the transfer of their sins onto it, at which time the animal was sacrificed as payment for their sins.

Now some of you may say that God is an all-loving God and wouldn't demand a price for forgiveness of sin. Yes, He is all-loving, but He is also a just God. He made the laws and when we break them, justice demands that a penalty be paid for breaking that law. (That is covered quite extensively in the sections regarding the natural-healing program.)

God made Jesus the ultimate sacrifice for all of us. From the day He died on the Cross, there was no need of any more animal sacrifice, so they ceased.

We are all sinners, but God made Jesus pay the penalty for our sins. We become a child of God by recognizing that He is the only way to God. In John 14:6 Jesus says, "I am the Way, the Truth and the Life. No one comes to the Father except through Me." Any attempt to get to God any other way is like saying to a judge that you will not pay the fine he imposes, but will pay what you want, when you want, and how you want. I don't think that would satisfy judgment for your crime. Anything we do to try to circumvent Christ is an insult to God and His creation. It's like spitting in His face.

Remember that when Jesus prayed in the Garden of Gethsemane, He asked the Father if there was any other way, to let this cup pass from Him. The "cup" He referred to was payment for our sins by His death, and His suffering our punishment in hell before He rose again. The fact that He submitted to the Cross tells me there was no other way, for He had the power to call forth the angels who would have stopped it instantly. He has all of heaven at His command. Even Satan attested to that when he tempted Jesus in the wilderness during His forty-day fast (see Matthew 4:5-6).

Ephesians 2:8-9 declares that "By grace are you saved, through faith. It is a gift of God, not of works, lest any man should boast." Yet a gift is only a gift if it is free. You can't earn it or buy it. The only way you can get it is, when it is offered, you reach out and take it. Until you do, it isn't yours. John 1:11-12 tells us, "He came to His own, and His own did not receive Him. But as many as received Him, to them He gave the right to become children of God, to those who believe in His name." And 1 John 5:11-12 affirms, "This is the testimony that God has given us eternal life, and this life is in His Son. He who has the Son has life; he who does not have the Son of God does not have life."

When we receive God's gift, Jesus' payment of our penalty for sin, then we are sealed with the Holy Spirit, the Third Person of the Trinity. What does that mean? Second Corinthians 1:21-22 assures us that "He who establishes us with you in Christ and has anointed us in God also has sealed us and given us the Spirit in our hearts as a guarantee."

So God is no longer outside us, trying to help us and draw us to Christ. But now He lives inside us in the Third Person of the Trinity, the Holy Spirit. That blows my mind that now, God Himself, LIVES INSIDE ME. Wow, if that doesn't change your life, I don't know what will.

It is the Spirit of God *inside* us that gives the power to break the chains of sin and addiction. Only God can break the bonds that hold us captive. Just like an apple tree will bear apples, so there will be changes in our lives as we allow the Holy Spirit to work in and through us as God's children. We are now rooted in God. We are a new tree, bearing different fruit.

Won't you ask Him to be your Savior and come into your heart today? He's worth it. If you need further help, we are here to help you. Just call 800-258-8589

Once you have accepted Christ as your Savior, the Holy Spirit dwells in you and 1 John 4:4 becomes true: "You are of God, little children, and have overcome them, because greater is He that is IN you than he that is in the world."

We all know of the existence of evil. We see it every day on the television and in the news. We hear about Satan worshipers, and the occult and its influence on children who sacrifice animals, and who even kill adults and babies. Prisons and mental hospitals are full of people who allowed Satan and demons to influence or possess them.

Refusing to accept Christ or trying to do it your own way is, in essence, choosing Satan's way, which results in choosing death. Remember, hell was prepared for Satan and his angels, the demons—and Satan is taking anyone with him who refuses to accept Christ.

When we stand before God at the judgment, He is going to look for one thing: IS OUR NAME WRITTEN DOWN IN THE BOOK OF LIFE AS HAVING RECEIVED

CHRIST? If not, then we will join Satan and his demons in hell. As Revelation 20:15 says, "Anyone not found written in the Book of Life was cast into the lake of fire." And when speaking of Heaven, Revelation 21:27 tells us, "There shall by no means enter in anything that defiles, or causes an abomination or a lie, but only those who are written in the Lamb's Book of Life."

Knowing what lies ahead for those who delve into the occult or Satan worship—and the havoc it brings—I ask *why* would anyone choose him or his ways over the wonderful, blessed peace that Christ offers? The first step in accepting Christ puts us in the place where we start the journey of healing and growth—it is the first "season" or baby step we must take.

The only way you will learn HOW to grow is to get into the Word of God. The Bible is His love letter to us, His instruction book on how to live the Christian life. First Peter 2:2 tenderly refers to new Christians as newborn babies in Christ, and encourages them to "desire the pure milk of the Word, that you may grow thereby." From there, we grow and change and find release. Second Timothy 2:15 calls us to be diligent in studying the Scriptures to present ourselves "approved to God, a worker who does not need to be ashamed, rightly dividing the Word of truth."

I love the bumper sticker that says, "Christians are not perfect, only forgiven." We are aligning ourselves with God's purpose for our life so we can fulfill all the wonderful things He has planned for us.

Over the years, I have had a few dealings with bad entities that were not pleasant, but I have seen God overcome in every instance. First and most important, good angels will always do things or tell you things that will line up with the Bible. Satan's angels, the demons (which are disembodied evil spirits) will not do that, but do everything they can to lead you astray or side-track you from God. They may even do "good" things or perform miracles, but their ultimate goal is deception and death to our souls.

Second Corinthians 11:13-14 warns us about people who are "false apostles, deceitful workers, transforming themselves into apostles of Christ. And no wonder! For Satan himself transforms himself into an angel of light." First John 4:1-3 says, "Beloved, do not believe every spirit, but test the spirits, whether they are of God, because many false prophets have gone out into the world. By this you know the Spirit of God: Every spirit that confesses that Jesus Christ has come in the flesh is of God, and every spirit that does not confess that Jesus Christ has come in the flesh is not of God."

The second way I can tell whether or not it is an angel or a bad spirit is by the way my own spirit responds. God doesn't scare us or play jokes on us. Every time I have had an encounter with an angel, there has always been a sense of peace. But if I am frightened or have an uncomfortable feeling in its presence, I know the spiritual being isn't coming from God. Second Timothy 1:7 assures us that "God has not given us a spirit of fear, but of power and of love and of a sound mind."

I don't believe evil spirits can take on a form, but either work unseen or possess something or someone. Angels can take on the form of a person or animal, whenever they need to, as they minister to mankind. This is evident in many of the accounts people relate of animals or people who showed up to rescue them and then vanished.

I'll tell you of some encounters I had with the bad ones first, and then leave you with some wonderful experiences. The incidents I will relate are from entities outside myself, which are different from the fears I experienced because of my own mind (such as my early fear of dead bodies).

The incident I related in Chapter 2 had to be a bad entity that took advantage of a sad emotional time because it created fear. God loves us—and we don't try to scare someone we love.

Well, after we left that house in North Argyle, bad entities never seemed to have any other influence on me until the spring of 1993 when I met with some people who claimed they had been abducted by UFOs. I began to believe them and became fascinated by their stories.

Gradually, I noticed subtle changes. I had always loved the night, taking long walks in the cool, star-studded quiet when the world was asleep. Seldom did I ever go to bed before 2 a.m., and when offered shifts in a job that required 24-hour-a-day attendants, I always chose the swing or night shift.

Yet I began to fear the onset of evening with its long, dark hours. Every night at 2 a.m., I suddenly became aware of the time and, when asleep, I was startled awake to see the hands on the clock standing out, greatly enlarged, as though the clock face was a neon sign. Balls of light darted around my darkened room. Items also started disappearing from the house such as a camera and an expensive soup tureen.

Often at night while watching TV, I became aware that two hours had suddenly passed (usually from 2 a.m. to 4 a.m.), and that the movie was over but I hadn't seen it. Yet I knew I hadn't fallen asleep.

One day I saw a video called "UFOs: The Mystery Resolved." It talked about the dynamics of UFOs being the same as demon activity, creating illusions as the laws of physics were being totally violated.

They suggested we approach the incidents as demonic activity. So I walked my twenty-acre property, binding and casting out Satan. I remember telling him that the things he took didn't belong to him, and that he'd better put them back because I belonged to God and everything I owned belonged to God.

Within minutes, the camera appeared where it had not been earlier, and the soup tureen was in the cupboard again. Now, several people who worked for me had spent *days* looking for that tureen, which hadn't been in the cupboard. But now, suddenly it was there.

When I started to feel fear as the night again approached, I told Satan, in Jesus' name, to get out and leave me alone, that he had no place in my life. Instantly the fear left, and the hands on the clock stopped standing out at 2 a.m.

The last of these incidents happened late one night. I was again awakened by balls of light darting around the room. Immediately I bound Satan and told him to quit trying to intimidate me. I didn't buy it anymore and he was being pretty obvious.

Once I realized what was happening and took a stand against the demons, all their harassment stopped. If they had been real UFOs from other planets, then it would have continued. Again, Satan frightens us, not God. And Satan can only win if you allow his intimidation to work. If you don't, he has to flee.

I'm not making a judgment of every experience people have had, just relating what happened to me. I don't know if there are beings on other planets. I wouldn't be surprised! Why not? Do we think that we are the only beings God created in this incredibly vast universe that we have only begun to explore or discover! My, how egotistical man can be.

ANGELS

I hear of so many people asking God to get rid of Satan. Yet some things, I believe, are put into the hands of believers to do. In Matthew 16:17-19, Jesus is talking to Peter and refers to Peter's confession that Jesus is the Christ, the Son of the living God. Jesus then gives to all those who also believe this, "the keys of the kingdom of heaven," and says, "Whatever you bind on earth will be bound in heaven and whatever you loose on earth, will be loosed in heaven."

James 4:7 tells us, "Submit to God. Resist the devil and he will flee from you." WE are to resist him and he will flee. Mark 16:17 and Matthew 10:1 affirm that Jesus gave His *followers* power to cast out unclean spirits in *His* Name—not in their own strength.

So if you don't know Christ, don't try casting out demons or telling them to go! Read the incident in Acts 19:13-16:

> Then some of the itinerant Jewish exorcists took it upon themselves to call the name of the Lord Jesus over those who had evil spirits, saying, "We exorcise you by the Jesus whom Paul preaches." Also there were seven sons of Sceva, a Jewish chief priest, who did so. And the evil spirit answered and said, "Jesus I know, and Paul I know; but who are you?" Then the man in whom the evil spirit was, leaped on them, overpowered them, and prevailed against them, so that they fled out of the house naked and wounded.

Some people joke about poltergeists, thinking they are playful spirits that just have a little fun with people. They will often let them dwell in their homes and laugh about their antics. I feel this is dangerous as either a spirit is a good angel or it is a demon. Nowhere in Scripture do I find playful spirits like poltergeists or Casper the friendly ghost. This may be a cute story for children, but is definitely not true.

Since Satan comes as an angel of light (or a seemingly fun spirit?), the ultimate end is destruction and devastation. I once met a "poltergeist" in Azusa, California, where a client was laughingly telling me she had one, as though it were some kind of pet or something. She would find candles lit on both ends, things moved around her house where she hadn't put them. Once before getting in the shower, she put her cigarette in an ashtray, and when she got out, it was lit on both ends.

When I showed her from Scripture that I thought it was dangerous to continue to entertain it, she decided maybe it was time it left. I walked through the house, praying and binding Satan and his demons, quoting Scripture to it. Several weeks later, she reported that it left that night and never came back.

There's one thing that's helpful when you are suspicious that you have a bad entity around you or in your home: Fill your house with Christ-centered praise music and Bible-reading tapes. Satan can't bear to live where Christ is honored.

One time I moved into a dog kennel that was absolutely filthy. It had been occupied by and surrounded by neighbors who were definitely not Christ-centered. I could feel a very heavy spirit there that I just couldn't shake. One day I was praying about how to get rid of it when I received the message to clean it up and, as I did, it would leave. An unclean spirit that could not dwell in order and peace had lived in that kennel. I remodeled the house and as I did, the "spirit" lifted.

Other problems such as illness and financial problems are not necessarily caused by demonic presence, although these things can be evil-inspired. (I have covered that concept in other chapters, so I will stick to our present topic.)

A client in Arcadia, California, asked me to come to her house to find out what was causing weird noises and items to move around on their own. Since her animals were also frightened, I went there, pretty sure I was dealing with evil entities. I fasted and prayed before I went, but no amount of exorcism removed the problem. In fact, nothing happened then or later. I couldn't understand what had happened, until several years later when I visited a "psychic healer" whose clients come to her home for "healing."

This is a very gracious, giving person, not one you would think was dealing with demons, but she is. She honestly believes she is working with God, but knowing her overall theology, I know that her mind has been blinded. I still pray for her often as I do love her as a person.

That day, I sat on her couch, holding my little dogs close and asking God for the protection and covering of the Blood of Jesus as she started "working" on her patient. Suddenly I felt a being brush past me. Immediately, I bound it and tried to cast it out. I was startled to "hear" a voice answer me. It was so clear and definitely not what I expected, so I know it wasn't my imagination. "You can't cast me out," it told me. "This is her home and she invited me in. But I can't touch you or your animals."

As I have since studied Scripture and the experiences of other people, I have come to realize that in every instance where Jesus or the disciples cast out demons, it was when that person came to them for deliverance. I realized that, in the above two cases, I couldn't exorcise them because I was in the home of a person who didn't want or recognize Christ as Savior.

In essence, even though they weren't consciously aware of working with or allowing the entrance of Satan and his demons into their lives or homes, they did just that. But *they* had to be the ones who wanted the demons to leave. I couldn't do that for them.

ONLY the person who has the Spirit of God dwelling in them, as believers in Christ, have the total protection of God when they walk in His will and in obedience to His Word.

This was brought home to me in an even clearer way when I lived in Duarte, California. It was soon after I received the baptism of the Holy Spirit and started communicating with animals, so I was pretty sensitive to His voice. My neighbor's husband was an alcoholic who had a very violent nature, and often abused and beat his family. I was sitting in my living room one afternoon, praying for them as I listened to his cursing and shouting.

Suddenly God spoke to me and said, *Get over there NOW. George is going to kill them.*

Now, I am not one to interfere. But in this instance, it was so strong that I jumped up, without even a second's hesitation, and ran for their backdoor, which was only about fifteen feet from mine. I threw open the door and yelled, "George, in the name of Jesus of Nazareth, I command you to leave your family alone!"

As he ran through the house to where I was standing at the backdoor, I yelled, "Mel, get Lisa and get over to my house!" When George arrived at the door, I saw that he had a metal pipe in his right hand and was furious. He raised his right arm and came at me with all the fury and strength he could muster. But an amazing thing happened. Suddenly, he couldn't move. His arm was suspended in midair and he couldn't move.

A shocked look flooded his face as he turned to look at his right arm, but no one was there. He grabbed it with his left hand and pulled with all his strength, but the right arm remained suspended midair as though someone were holding it.

ANGELS

I didn't move or say another word until I heard Mel and Lisa enter my front door. Then I quietly let go of the door and walked back to my house. As I started through my backdoor, I looked back at George. He just stood there, eyes staring at me, silent as a statue.

The instant I put my foot through my door, his arm dropped and he fell forward: The force or angel who held him had let him go, and he plummeted down the steps with the momentum that matched the strength he had applied to pull himself free.

In this incident, God used me to save Mel's and Lisa's life, and an angel to save mine. Previously, when I had tried to talk to George about accepting Christ as Savior, he had become angry. From that time on, whenever he saw me, he crossed to the other side of the street to avoid me. Never again did I see him harm his family when he knew I was home. Within a few short months, Mel, who was one of the sweetest ladies I have ever known, died of a heart attack. George later got hit by a car and killed while crossing a street.

But the saddest of all is Lisa. She got married to get out of the house and away from her father—only to find that her husband was as abusive and more dangerous than her father had been. She knows that her husband will kill her if she tries to leave, so she is trapped in an even worse situation, with two little boys to care for. This seems to happen so often. I wonder if this isn't part of what God was talking about when He said the sins of the parents are visited on the children. In this case, it sure seems like it.

Be careful what you read or allow in your home. That can cause you such problems! You might think you're sick or having mental problems, but it may just be what you have allowed in with those items. Children are particularly susceptible to harassment from demonic spirits. You must get rid of those items—books, whatever. Denounce them, ask God's forgiveness for your involvement with them, and fill your house with praise and worship to Christ. Then the demons will leave, if you know the Lord. But if you don't know Him, you'd better get right with Him so you can enjoy the kind of protection I've talked about in this chapter.

Never, never, never allow your children to play with Ouija boards—or even allow the boards in your house. If you do, you are opening your home to demonic spirits. It is not a game, and most children know there is something in that board. We had two experiences that proved it.

One night a Christian friend of mine, who was married to a man preparing for ministry at Bible college, visited friends who were playing with a Ouija board. She warned them that it was dangerous, but they didn't believe her. She then proceeded to prove it by putting her hands on the board. The pointer, called a planchette, kept going off the board. Finally she asked the board why, and it spelled out "Because you love Jesus." When that happened, everyone in the room became frightened, so they gathered up everything to do with it, and threw it into the fireplace. As it burned, it screamed.

One time, I visited a client who was working a Ouija board when I arrived. She asked me to sit down and do it with her, but I refused. She told me she used it every day, and never went out of the house without asking it for advice and help.

Now, she had called me in to find out why her young son had started having nightmares. When I told her I believed that the spirit in the board was responsible, she laughed. To prove it to her, I sat down and began asking it questions.

At first, the planchette tried not to move for me, but kept trying to go off the board. When I asked it why, it spelled out "church." Then I asked it, "In the name of Jesus, I command you to tell me, what is your name?" It replied by spelling out "Lying Spirit." I again demanded, "In the name of Jesus, where did you come from?" to which it replied, "hell."

At that point, she destroyed the "game," denounced it, and together we walked through the house and prayed. The child's nightmares stopped from then on, as did the sounds of knocking on his wall that had also been occurring nightly.

At one time, I had attended some "psychic" fairs and had become interested in automatic writing. One night, I decided to try it. I had always had trouble making changes in my life of any kind, so I asked my subconscious why. It replied, "Because of an unmovable mother." Well, that made sense to me because my mother was very rigid, never changing her standards. OK, that was profitable.

But then I started thinking about the Scripture that tells us to "try the spirits whether they are of God" (1 John 4:1). So I started asking questions.

"Is your body alive?"

Answer: "No."

"Where did you live when you were alive?"

Reply: "Armenia."

"What do you want?"

Reply: "May I enter you?"

I was totally freaked! I dropped the pen and yelled, "No! In the name of Jesus I bind you and command you to go back where you came from!" I quickly repented, denounced it, and never tried automatic writing again.

I definitely don't ever recommend you step in harm's way, like I did, unless you are absolutely certain God is telling you to. As long as you are in His will, He will protect you with whatever He tells you to do. But when we step out on our own strength or out of His will, disobedience opens us to possible attack.

Unfortunately, I learned that lesson the hard way.

One time I was on a lecture tour, heading for a retrieving-dog training kennel and teaching facility to conduct a seminar. As I left Dallas and headed south, a feeling of apprehension grew stronger and stronger. I knew that God was telling me not to go there, but I couldn't "see" a logical reason not to, so I went.

It was a disaster, and I am joyful to say it won't happen again because I have now learned to do what He indicates and not just listen to what I perceive as logic. I ended up staying there one week because my back went out and I was down in bed. When I was finally able to get up and move, the further I got from there, the better my back felt.

Another time I was driving south on Highway 1, near the border between Oregon and California, when I became very tired. I pulled over into what looked like a nice, quiet place to camp. I had three German Shepherds, trained to protect, so I wasn't afraid to be alone in the woods. But as I pulled the bed down in my camper, took the dogs for a walk and prepared to stay, the same feeling of apprehension came over me. With each passing minute, it became stronger and stronger, with pictures of people surrounding my camper, smashing the windows with axes and clubs, and bludgeoning us to death. I couldn't get out of there fast enough, and even though I was tired and sleepy, didn't stop for the night until the fear had passed. I don't know what happened back there, but I am sure glad I didn't find out.

I'm sure many of you can relate similar experiences, and many more. But let me share with you the pièce de résistance: my experiences of how God saved my life and protected those I love.

ANGELS

It happened the first time within a couple of weeks of our arrival in Sarasota, Florida, when I was 14 years old. We stayed at a trailer park on Siesta Key, just south of town. Oh, what a wonderful place that was, on the bay with the Gulf of Mexico right across the street.

Every afternoon, as soon as Yvonne and I got off the school bus, we headed for the beach. Now, for water-lover Bea, a very accomplished swimmer who had grown up on lakes and rivers, the warm water of the gulf was paradise. Yvonne didn't swim well, but for this water bug it was truly a time to rejoice. Never having dealt with tides before, I always assumed that waves came into shore and deposited everything onto the beach. So I felt safe, floating and snoozing to their gentle rhythm.

One afternoon, I must have fallen asleep while the tide was going out. I don't have any idea how long I slept, but when I awoke and tried to stand up, there was no bottom and I could barely see the shoreline. I was really scared because I'd heard a lot of shark stories, but I also didn't doubt my ability to swim to shore.

But as I started back, I realized I was unaware of how waves worked. With every few strokes, another wave would knock me under. All of a sudden, I heard a man's gentle voice telling me how to swim with the waves, instead of fighting them. I told him I was scared my parents would kill me if anything happened to my little sister, so I had to hurry because I couldn't see her from there. "She's fine," he replied. "I can see her playing in the sand."

It never dawned on me to question why a stranger, who looked to be in his 50s, was at least a mile out in the Gulf of Mexico and swimming right next to me. We only took a few strokes and instantly, with no sensation of it happening, we were at shore.

I stood up, looked at Yvonne, then turned back to thank him, and he was gone. I remember being a little puzzled because it was a large, open beach with no place to hide. And since I had only turned away for two seconds, he couldn't have gotten out of sight that fast!

I know now that he was an angel sent to rescue me. This was the first time I had seen one, and it wasn't until years later that I fully realized what had happened.

The next time, I didn't see the angel, but felt it. I was 16 years old and had just gotten my drivers license two months previously. My stepbrother Ben had been in an automobile accident, so Mom flew to New York to be with him, while the rest of us followed by car.

Dad, Yvonne and I were driving north along old, slow, winding roads (this was before super highways like Interstate 75). My dad had driven so long that he was tired, so he decided to let me drive while he got some sleep in the back seat.

He hadn't been sleeping long when suddenly the right-front tire blew out. We were going at a pretty good speed, around a curve that, if unchecked, would have pulled us right off the road into a ditch.

I FROZE, barely touching the steering wheel. I didn't know what to do since the driving manuals didn't address this type of situation. Suddenly I felt a "force" come over my body and hands, the wheel quickly turned the car back on the road (the opposite of what it would have done), and the brake pressed to the floor, stopping the car. Well, the phenomenon of suddenly being moved, without experiencing any sensation of it, left me feeling quite incredulous. Satan may have tried to kill us, but again, God intervened.

Something like that happened again on a dark, rainy night when I was heading home on the San Bernardino Freeway, near

Temple City, California. I was going about forty miles per hour when I suddenly realized a massive pileup was occurring in my lane just ahead. There wasn't enough time to slip into the next lane, which was already filled with cars anyway. So I called out the name of Jesus, over and over.

I never moved the wheel and never felt the movement, but the next thing I knew, I was in the outside lane, safely going past the lanes of piled-up cars. I was filled with wonder at what had just happened, and praised God for His deliverance as I drove safely home.

I had a similar experience with my animals on Highway 101 when I was heading home after a trip to San Francisco. By now, I am sure you know how important my animals are to me. I always have them with me in the motor home for company and protection. We had been traveling for a few hours when I noticed they were restless and needed to get out for a pit stop. I found a dirt road and pulled several yards back behind the fence that blocked it from the freeway. The three dogs I had with me were always obedient, returning when they were called, so I let them run without leashes.

Out of nowhere a rabbit appeared, sat up in front of them until they noticed it, and took off running for the freeway. Well, if you know anything about rabbit behavior, you'll know that they don't stop to sit up in front of a pack of dogs until they're noticed. Instead, rabbits run to their hole where they are safe— and *not* to a busy freeway.

My dogs had often chased rabbits down their hole and proceeded to make fools of themselves, digging frantically trying to find that rabbit. Meanwhile, the rabbit had traveled through his tunnel, and now sat on a mound a good distance away, watching their ridiculous antics. This rabbit's behavior was so out of character for rabbits, for *this one* headed straight for the freeway.

It was then that I knew I was dealing with a spiritual entity intent on destroying what was most important to me: my dogs and foundation breeding stock.

No matter how I called, my dogs were bent on catching that rabbit. Next I watched in horror, crying out the Name of Jesus over and over, as they tore through a barbed-wire fence and headed straight in front of an enormous tractor-trailer speeding down the highway. Until that moment, I had always known that God loved me and would protect me, but I always wondered if He would protect my beloved animals.

I am so grateful He had another miracle in store for me.

As my dogs started across the road, the tractor-trailer descended on them going at least sixty miles per hour. I saw the truck *begin* to drive over the first two—and then they vanished. Then I saw the third one begin to run *through* the front tires. But suddenly, she wasn't there, either. And no bodies were thrown anywhere!

When the truck passed, my dogs stood quietly on the center divider, looking about in a dazed manner. With cars whizzing by, they walked calmly back across three lanes of traffic. Not one vehicle attempted to avoid them or applied its brakes and yet, when I looked them over, the only scratch on them was the one Philea had gotten on her chest when she went through the barbed wire.

I know I saw them go through that truck. Not under it, *through* it—much like how Thomas saw Jesus enter the room in John 20:26.

I don't know how to explain it, but it happened. Without God's intervention (and His angels?), I would not have had my three-foundation breeding stock, my friends. Through the years, many more friends came from them—some of which are still with me today. I am so grateful. Life has not been easy, but

I am glad I serve a God who loves me the way He has demonstrated time and time again.

Remember, as in Job's case and many others, Satan can only get away with what God allows Him to. He can and will intimidate us, but can only defeat us if we give him the power to do so by believing that intimidation.

When I was writing the booklet, "How to Cope With the Death of a Pet," I experienced that intimidation and harassment quite often. But God never allowed Satan to win. Many times, I would enter something in my word processor, and run off a copy so I could edit it later. The next day, I would attempt to retrieve it, only to find out it was erased. I'd then start looking for the printed copy, only to find that it, too, was gone from the top of the processor, where I had put it the night before. Eventually I would find it, re-enter it, and the same process would begin again.

Nothing else got erased or "misplaced." Only that booklet.

Things finally came to a head when I searched my writing room for the copy, but to no avail. The booklet had been nearly completed, down to the final draft. But it was no longer in the computer's memory, and my hard copy was gone.

After a frustrating couple of hours, I finally stopped, realizing this was an attempt by Satan to stop the booklet's completion. So I took the authority of the Word and bound Satan, demanding that he release it back to me. Instantly, I felt a strong urge to go look in the motor home. Logic kept arguing with me, telling me it couldn't be there as I hadn't been to the motor home for days—especially since I had last worked on the booklet. But what did I have to lose? Nothing but a few minutes.

So I looked. And there it was, laying on the bed in the back of the motor home. From that day on, it never disappeared again.

I am often asked to communicate with dead animals and people. I do not do this as it is forbidden in the Bible. In 1 Samuel 28, Saul had purged the land of mediums because it was one of God's commands from Leviticus 20:27: "A man or a woman who is a medium or who has familiar spirits shall surely be put to death; they shall stone them with stones. Their blood shall be upon them."

Yes, it is possible to call up the dead as Scripture seems to indicate. But as recorded in Isaiah 8:19: "When they say to you, 'Seek those who are mediums and wizards, who whisper and mutter,' should not a people seek their God? Should they seek the dead on behalf of the living?"

They can't help you anymore, and because they have passed over doesn't automatically make them omniscient (all-knowing). Remember the account in Luke 16 where Jesus told the parable that taught the truth that once a person has passed on, there is a great gulf between them. Even though the dead may want to send messages back, God forbids it. In verses 30 and 31 of this parable, a rich man (who had died) asks Abraham to send Lazarus (also dead) to the rich man's family because "'If one goes to them from the dead, they will repent.' But Abraham said to him, 'If they do not hear Moses and the prophets, neither will they be persuaded though one rise from the dead.'"

You never know to whom or to what you are talking because that is a realm you cannot "see" to identify. The only safe spirit or spirit guide you can talk to is the Holy Spirit of God. First Timothy 2:5 tells us that "There is one God and one Mediator between God and men, the Man Christ Jesus."

And in John 16:13-16, Jesus assures us, "When He, the Spirit of truth, has come, He will guide you into all truth; for He will not speak on His own authority, but whatever He hears He will speak; and He will tell you things to come. He will glorify Me, for He will take of what is Mine and declare it to you. All things that the Father has are Mine. Therefore, I said that He will take of Mine and declare it to you."

The Holy Spirit will never deceive us, but will lead us into all truth. He will always be there for us, and may call down God's ministering angels to protect us. But we are not to pray to the angels directly or ask them for help, and they don't speak through us.

But as we look to the Lord and pray, as Daniel did, God sends them.

And who knows? Maybe one day you too may ...

... Meet or entertain an angel unaware.